INVISIBLE ILLNESS

The publisher and the University of California Press Foundation gratefully acknowledge the generous support of the Barbara S. Isgur Endowment Fund in Public Affairs.

INVISIBLE ILLNESS

A History, from Hysteria to Long COVID

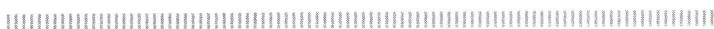

EMILY MENDENHALL

UNIVERSITY OF CALIFORNIA PRESS

University of California Press
Oakland, California

Library of Congress Cataloging-in-Publication Data

Names: Mendenhall, Emily, 1982- author
Title: Invisible illness : a history, from hysteria to long Covid / Emily
    Mendenhall.
Description: Oakland, California : University of California Press, [2026] |
    Includes bibliographical references and index.
Identifiers: LCCN 2025019105 (print) | LCCN 2025019106 (ebook) | ISBN
    9780520421523 cloth | ISBN 9780520421530 ebook
Subjects: LCSH: Chronic diseases—United States—History | Hysteria—United
    States—History | Post COVID-19 condition (Disease)—United
    States--History | Chronically ill—Care—Social aspects—United States |
    People with disabilities—Care—Social aspects—United States |
    Discrimination in medical care—United States—History | Medical
    anthropology--United States
Classification: LCC RA644.6 .M46 2026 (print) | LCC RA644.6 (ebook) |
    DDC 616/.0478—dc23/eng/20250730
LC record available at https://lccn.loc.gov/2025019105
LC ebook record available at https://lccn.loc.gov/2025019106

Manufactured in the United States of America

GPSR Authorized Representative: Easy Access System Europe, Mustamäe tee 50,
10621 Tallinn, Estonia, gpsr.requests@easproject.com

35   34   33   32   31   30   29   28   27   26
10   9   8   7   6   5   4   3   2   1

For Peter

Contents

A Note on Names

MANY PEOPLE FEEL MORE COMFORTABLE sharing intimate details of their lives under a pseudonym. For two decades I've spent hours listening to people share their narratives of chronic illness and in doing so feel some relief or perhaps liberty through their anonymity. This project, while surprising for many reasons, was unexpected because of the extent to which many people wanted the opposite: they wanted their names to be unabashedly displayed. Upon their requests, I use the real names of most people whose stories are central to this book. However, there are some people who do not feel safe sharing their names, either because they believe it will impinge on their ability to get a job or they fear people will discriminate against them in other ways, and have asked me to conceal their identity. I indicate throughout the book when a name is a pseudonym. When someone's story is shared in great depth, the story has been reviewed and approved, with revisions, through several drafts until both of us are happy with how it is crafted, the content shared, and what is conveyed.

A Glossary of Conditions

||||||||||||||||||||||||||||||||||||||||||||||||||||||||||||||||||||||||||||||||||||||||||||||||||||||||||||||||||||||||||||||||||||||||||||||||||||||||||||||||||||||||||||||||||||||

BEFORE WE GET STARTED, I put together a glossary for the complex chronic health conditions that appear throughout the book for you to review, reconcile, and remember which conditions are which, how they are diagnosed, and what they do in the bodymind. I use the crip term *bodymind* to reflect the inherent intersectional interrelatedness of mind and body; in this way, I am talking about the mind and body as an integrated whole as opposed to separate entities. *Crip* refers to the disability justice movement and the ways in which people living with disabling conditions reclaim words and concepts to serve as empowering sources.[1]

This glossary is not an exhaustive list, nor is it a comprehensive or definitive one. I define these health conditions by their complexity and the trouble they cause in diagnosis, lived experience, treatment, care, and recovery. However, I list these descriptions while also knowing that most people have one *primary* diagnosis in addition to one or more secondary diagnoses. This is one reason people with the same diagnosis do not always experience the same symptoms or course of illness. Yet, most people experience one or more flagship symptoms, such as muscle weakness, disabling fatigue, post-exertional malaise exacerbation, headaches, dizziness and trouble standing for long periods, memory inconsistency, brain fog, light sensitivity, numbness of the fingers and toes, chronic pain, hallucination, and psychological distress (like panic, anxiety, and depression). Most people have a unique cluster of symptoms that may also accompany other chronic conditions, such as autoimmune diseases, diabetes, heart disease, cancers, and others.

I constructed these definitions based on a combination of readings from the US National Institutes of Health as well as #MEpedia, a project of #MEAction (a patient activist organization). I chose the first source because of its broad scientific impact and legitimacy as a medical organization. I chose the second source because it is a patient-led organization that works together to elevate and advise research, promote public education, and provide patients living with complex chronic conditions a community of support and knowledge. I also received feedback on these definitions from several scholars and activists living with chronic illnesses.

ANKYLOSING SPONDYLITIS is a type of arthritis that causes inflammation in the joints and ligaments of the spine, sometimes affecting the peripheral joints like the knees, ankles, and hips.

CHRONIC FATIGUE is a general term used to relay conditions that cause general fatigue but is not considered a diagnostic category. Many patients find clinical use of this term problematic.

CHRONIC FATIGUE SYNDROME (CFS) was defined by the Centers for Disease Control and Prevention in 1994 by the Fukuda criteria; it was a common diagnosis in the 1990s and 2000s and remains common in the southern United States and United Kingdom. It is a broad category of symptoms, including chronic fatigue but also several symptoms characterized by dysautonomia.

COMPLEX REGIONAL PAIN SYNDROME (CRPS) is a form of pain that affects the arms or legs, often after a surgery, stroke, or heart attack, which is out of proportion to the severity of the initial injury.

DYSAUTONOMIA is caused when the autonomic nervous system fails to regulate the brain, heart, blood, and gut. It manifests differently between people and produces common symptoms like heart palpitations, memory inconsistency, sensitivity to sound and light, dizziness and problems with balance, low blood sugar, sweating, diarrhea, chest pain, migraines, and mood swings. Rarely are two people's experiences the same: dysautonomia often appears in conjunction with and accompanies other complex chronic conditions.

DYSTONIA is a movement disorder where the muscles contract involuntarily, sometimes causing repetitive or twisting movements either in one part of the bodymind (focal dystonia), two or more connected parts of the bodymind (segmental dystonia), or the whole bodymind (general dystonia).

ENDOMETRIOSIS is a reproductive condition where lining of the uterus travels, and tissues are found on the reproductive organs or sometimes beyond. This causes heavy bleeding and extraordinary abdominal pain.

EPSTEIN-BARR VIRUS (EBV, also known as human herpesvirus 4) is a common human virus associated with mononucleosis, which spreads through saliva and other bodily fluids. It's very contagious and stays (often dormant) in the bodymind forever. EBV can be associated with chronic ear infections and diarrhea in children and with severe conditions in adults, like Guillain-Barre syndrome and certain cancers. It's theorized that EBV couples with other viruses (like SARS-CoV-2) and causes more severe and disabling symptoms.

FIBROMYALGIA is a chronic and persistent disorder that causes pain and tenderness throughout the bodymind. The condition has been theorized to result from inflammation of the fascia, which is intramuscular connective tissue that runs throughout the bodymind, is richly innervated, and is known to secrete inflammatory proteins (like cytokines).[2]

FUNCTIONAL NEUROLOGICAL DISORDER (FND) is a psychiatric diagnosis also known as conversion disorder or somatoform disorder. FND is diagnosed when there is no apparent structural damage but the patient experiences several unexplained symptoms. (It's often quipped as a software problem as opposed to a hardware problem). FND can be a contentious diagnosis for patients who have unverifiable conditions and believe there may be viral or bacterial origins.

GASTROPARESIS is a condition where there is immense stomach pain when food doesn't empty properly and causes a solid mass called a bezoar. These are often caused by viral infections or lifelong metabolic conditions like diabetes.

HYPERMOBILE EHLERS-DANLOS SYNDROME (hEDS) is a connective tissue disorder that affects the structure of collagen throughout the bodymind, though its precise cause is unknown. It is a subset of a broader condition called Ehlers-Danlos syndrome, which involves several subtypes.

HYSTERIA was a common medical condition in the nineteenth and twentieth centuries, characterizing neurological symptoms that were exaggerated or inappropriately emotional. The condition was associated with the nervous system and the womb, and many perceived it to be functional (or psychological) in nature.

LONG COVID is an infection-associated chronic condition that is an umbrella term for any illness after a COVID-19 infection. It may include biological vulnerability of the heart, lungs, kidneys, blood, and other organs; it is often associated with dysregulation of the autonomic nervous system. Many people diagnosed with long COVID have symptom profiles that are closely aligned with dysautonomia.

LUPUS, OR SYSTEMIC LUPUS ERYTHEMATOSUS (SLE), is a chronic autoimmune condition that attacks the bodymind's own tissues, causing inflammation and in some cases permanent tissue damage. It's perniciously systemic and hard to identify; symptoms resemble dysautonomia.

LYME DISEASE develops from a corkscrew-shaped bacterium called a spirochete (known as *Borrelia burgdorferi*) that is carried by ticks; when this bacterium is released from the tick, it moves into the blood and eventually travels to the brain and is often identified by a red scaly rash that looks like a bullseye or solid-colored lesion. The chronic condition resembles dysautonomia.

MAST CELL ACTIVATION SYNDROME (MCAS) is a condition that causes mast cells to release an inappropriate amount of chemicals into the bodymind. When the chemical histamine is released, it may cause extreme allergy symptoms, including itchy and swollen skin, expanding blood vessels, mucus buildup, headaches, wheezing, and trouble breathing.

MÉNIÈRE'S DISEASE is a form of dysautonomia and balance disorder that is caused by an abnormality in the labyrinth, which is part of the inner ear. Flare-ups may cause vertigo, as well as hearing loss. For some it causes tinnitus.

MYALGIC ENCEPHALOMYELITIS (ME) is a condition coined by Melvin Ramsey, a doctor who responded to the Royal Free Hospital outbreak in London in 1954, and is defined by the International Consensus Criteria for ME. It closely resembles dysautonomia.

MYALGIC ENCEPHALOMYELITIS/CHRONIC FATIGUE SYNDROME (ME/CFS) is a condition designated in 2004 by the Canadian Consensus Criteria. It is an infection-associated chronic condition that is immune-mediated but affects multiple systems of the bodymind, from the central and autonomic nervous systems to the immune, cardiovascular, endocrine, digestive, and musculoskeletal systems. It closely resembles dysautonomia and is sometimes diagnosed with fibromyalgia. It is a more widely used (and preferred) diagnosis than ME, CFS, or chronic fatigue. Some people with long COVID also identify with ME/CFS.

NEURASTHENIA is an outdated neurological condition characterized by weakness of the physical nerves. It was largely perceived, much like hysteria, to be functional (psychological). Although hysteria was largely (but not exclusively) linked to women, neurasthenia was associated with combat veterans (who were often men) as well as nonveterans who were men or women. Many people presenting with neurasthenia showed symptoms of dysautonomia.

POSTURAL ORTHOSTATIC TACHYCARDIA SYNDROME (POTS) is a circulatory disorder where blood stays in the lower bodymind when someone stands up, and in response, the heart rate escalates. Changing positions causes the orthostatic intolerance, causing symptoms like dizziness, lightheadedness, nausea, blurred vision, pain, bloating, diarrhea or constipation, and vomiting.

SEPTAD is the name used, especially among patients and some physicians, to refer to a Venn diagram of several often-overlapping conditions. Many people are diagnosed with autoimmune conditions, such as Sjögren's syndrome or lupus, or connective tissue disorders like hypermobile Ehlers-Danlos syndrome. Many develop mast cell activation syndrome (MCAS) and dysautonomia or postural orthostatic tachycardia syndrome (POTS). Others have infections from Epstein-Barr virus or Coxsackie B4 or illnesses such as Lyme disease, ME/CFS, or long COVID. Many have gastric issues, such as gastroparesis or small intestinal bacterial overgrowth. Others demonstrate structural anomalies associated with the brain and spine.[3]

SJÖGRENS SYNDROME is an autoimmune disease where the immune system attacks its own tissues; while there appears to be a genetic component, viruses and bacteria may trigger the condition. It's usually recognized when mucous membranes and moisture-secreting glands of the eyes and mouth are affected and cause a reduction in tears and saliva (causing dry eyes and mouth). It often develops alongside rheumatoid arthritis and lupus.

INTRODUCTION

QUARANTINE WAS ABOUT TO BEGIN in Portland. A longtime customer stopped by Bethany McCraw's salon just as she was readying to close for the night. She was exhausted but needed the money. What could it hurt to do one more haircut before the world shut down?, she thought. Halfway through the cut, her customer said anxiously, "I think I might have it!" Bethany—a quirky artist who'd worked in high-end fashion around the world—stepped back and listened intently. His mother lived in a COVID-19 hot spot and very recently died of "pneumonia." A week later his uncle died too. At the two funerals, everyone was coughing. The young man had only been back from the funerals for a few days. It was only on that day when he finally felt well enough to leave the house.

Bethany's symptoms started three days later. Bethany became one of many long COVID patients who never had a positive test after her acute symptoms first set in.[1] Tests weren't available that early in the pandemic in Oregon, and the hospitals were flooded with patients. When she called the emergency room, a nurse told her she didn't sound sick enough to come. "Stay home!" she said. "The emergency room is too crowded." Bethany stayed home to navigate shocking symptoms that kept her bedbound: high fevers, seizure-like spasms, dreamlike hallucinations, and stomach pains. She hacked so much she felt her throat close and her lungs close in. Her muscles started to intensively spasm, and she had trouble walking.

Ten days after the symptoms started, Bethany finally saw a doctor. The doctor's office had received their very first COVID-19 tests that morning, and she was the first person to be tested in their clinic. The man who tested her was holding her hand because she was pleading, "Am I really going to die?" He was in a full hazmat suit and looked at her through his goggles. But the results came a few days later: negative.

"Impossible," she thought. For weeks, she collapsed every time she stood up. She lost thirty pounds in the first twenty days of symptoms. Her hair matted and frizzed. She had rashes all over her skin. Her fingers and toes turned blue. Her gums bled. Her teeth broke from grinding. "I know I had it," she said to me. "What else could it be? I've never been so sick in all my life." I nodded, remembering that she was a cancer survivor in her midfifties. Although cancer was a verifiable condition with a clear diagnosis and treatment plan, this was something else. Like millions of people around the world, Bethany began the arduous journey of an unverifiable, undiagnosed, unrecognized, untreated long-hauler, months before the term was even coined.

The first four months were brutal. Fever hit her like a truck. Bethany had spasms that presented like seizures. She was coughing up blood. Sometimes when she went to lie down, her arms, legs, and torso would jerk so much, she felt possessed. She would roll over in bed, flopping like a fish, unable to control her arms and legs. "And all I could do was just try to breathe through it. I had terrible fever, terrible dreams, and frightening hallucinations."

Bethany may have been frightened by her post-viral symptoms because, at first, she didn't understand them. This had not been the case with cancer. After a long career working in global elite hair design circuits, Bethany left that life to fulfill a lifelong dream of having a studio of her own. She restored an old Victorian home, outfitted a custom hair studio on the first floor, and remodeled the top two floors to live in. A thriving community of artists, friends, and clients found their way to her shop, and business boomed. She'd work twelve- to fourteen-hour days, welcoming stragglers in at all hours, shutting the lights off just before midnight. This life changed, a little over a year after she first opened, when she was diagnosed with breast cancer. In fact, it wasn't long after she'd recovered from breast cancer when she got COVID-19 for the first time.

When she first got sick from COVID-19, Bethany's friends would call her, but she was physically incapable of responding. In her head she would string together several cogent thoughts, but they could not exit her mouth. Her friends eventually stopped calling. A couple of months later her father died—he was the one family member with whom she had remained close. She felt that the trauma of these losses on top of her sickness was too much. She experienced some of her darkest days.

The loneliness was possibly the hardest part. She had no one to pick up groceries or help her organize and take her meds, prepare food, or take her to the doctor. She explained, "At that point I had no one . . . no family, no medical support, and my doctor told me it was all psychological. I didn't understand it. None of us did." In many ways, she felt what disabled activist Joanna Hedva has described on their philosophical blog *Sick Woman Theory* as "disposable."[2]

Some of the most startling experiences for many people living with long COVID are disruptions to cognition and memory. Bethany would move through some days in a trance. For example, she remembers sitting at her desk one day. Then suddenly she was in the kitchen and had no recollection of how she got there. This was the most severe of the few lapses she experienced, but the fact they occurred at all terrified her. "It felt like it wasn't me," she said. "It was like someone else had taken over my whole existence. I didn't know my own body or mind anymore." Her night-owl schedule flipped into a mornings-only routine. Most days she couldn't stay awake past 3 or 4 p.m. Some days she slept more than twenty-two hours in a stretch.

Most clinicians were unfamiliar with her symptoms and flummoxed by what to do: some would shrug and suggest she change her diet and lose weight. It absolutely infuriated her because her symptoms just got worse. However, the clinicians might have been as infuriated as she was; they had limited understanding of *why* she was suffering so much, with *what*, and *how* to help her.

During that first year of sickness, Bethany was unable to progress with her disability claims and had trouble getting any medical care at all. She was exhausted, and due to her severe migraines and brain fog, Bethany couldn't organize her case. "The disability access laws," she said, "suggested I should have gone in sooner." She found it difficult to sit upright, stand, climb the stairs between the three floors of her home, clean, or shower and dress herself. Her house fell into disarray. She felt abandoned not only by her family and friends but also by the state. She almost lost her house—until an attorney got involved.

The salon was still closed, and Bethany was broke. This meant she finally could access Medicaid and gain better access to health care. Bethany found a functional medical doctor who believed her symptoms were real, even if they didn't make complete sense to him. He diagnosed her with long COVID based on her symptoms, and they started tests that would unveil a great deal of information about her current symptoms. Bethany found him through a Facebook long COVID support group, based on a member's recommendation. In many ways, the virtual community had become the most reliable one in her life, often serving as the only people who believed her symptoms were real or could offer ideas about how to manage or reduce her pain.

They cogenerated what disability activist Mia Mingus has described as "access intimacy," where people with shared symptoms exchange social and emotional support and build legitimacy.[3] For many people, these relationships bring understanding and relief because they are recognized as living with a disabling condition—often for the first time. Bethany deeply valued the friends she met there. The new doctor ordered a whole slew of diagnostic testing that had been withheld before when clinicians were uncertain whether she really could have what she imagined.

Bethany's tests revealed that the virus had disrupted multiple systems at once. Her blood was sick. Her gut was off balance. Her inflammation markers were high. They discovered she had sleep apnea and worsening asthma and was prone to opportunistic secondary infections from fungus, like mold or yeast—all linked to the worsening condition of her house, which she was too weak to clean. Her immune function could not handle it all. She was diagnosed with postural orthostatic tachycardia syndrome, or POTS, a form of dysautonomia (when the autonomic nervous system becomes dysregulated), which affects functioning of the heart, gut, bladder, pupils, and blood.[4] These are not mildly acute symptoms, but things like disabling fatigue, dizziness, memory inconsistency, chronic muscular pain, and insomnia that upend a life by dysregulating the whole bodymind. Here, I use the word *bodymind*, as opposed to *mind* and/or *body*, to emphasize how the mind and body are deeply integrated and "tend to act as one".[5]

Most clinicians who read Bethany's case will find it dizzying. *What* is behind these befuddling symptoms? *Why* do things keep getting worse? *How* can we figure out ways to help her? In medicine, there is a tendency to push toward clarity, pinpointing exactly what is driving a physical symptom so that it might be rectified. This matters in part because ideas of unity and objectivity in science and medicine push against the tradition of thinking about complexity. As an anthropologist, I actively engage with a controversial set of mediators that may obscure stark divisions between fact and fiction, nature and nurture, truths and non-truths.[6] By interrogating truth claims in biomedicine, such as thinking about the body in terms of specificity—where there is an acute problem that must be fixed—I attempt to contextualize the bodymind in time and space and consider how people's political and family histories, relationships, and everyday lives might get under the skin.[7] In the case of Bethany, for example, part of her suffering involved a tremendous piling on of factors in her life and illness that pushed her over a *threshold*.

I use the metaphor of thresholds to explain the way many small vulnerabilities might build up until someone's combination of factors creates imbalance.[8] For instance, it might be that for some people a viral infection pushes them over a threshold into a corporeal imbalance, pushing the autonomic nervous system out of kilter and reverberating through multiple systems at once. However, the problem is never that one infection. Instead, these exposures might be tied to multiple insults, from family histories, mold and chemicals, metabolic irregularities in the blood, and previous viruses and bacteria that stay dormant and may reactivate in the nerves, gut, tissues, and brain. It is also our social histories, and traumatic experiences in particular, that become imprinted on and can wear down our immune, nervous, and digestive systems.[9] Concepts like weathering and allostatic load explain part of this and are central to understanding the thresholds metaphor. Weathering theorizes how cumulative threats wear down the immune system.[10] Allostatic load similarly may be understood as a tipping point when multiple systems dysregulate because the bodymind has been pushed to the brink.[11] In this way, thresholds are both temporal and corporeal—they are the moment equilibrium becomes disrupted, and interdependence breaks down, causing a slow and prolonged unraveling of multiple systems.

"COVID is like lighter fluid, an igniter, and is a simmering underlying flame," Monica Verduzco-Gutierrez, a physician and researcher who has now lived with long COVID for several years, told me. I met her at a meeting at the National Academies and followed up with her for an interview. She explained, "It is the lighter fluid, and it brings whatever is existing out." This theory may explain why so many people present in varied ways: the virus exacerbates whatever underlying conditions are already there. It might be that you have a propensity for anxiety, and the virus spins it out of control. Or that there is an underlying heart condition that has not yet reared its fiery head, but the virus wakes it up. Or you have an autoimmune condition that hasn't been diagnosed, but you find it when you're seeking care for more severe symptoms.[12] "It's like unpeeling an onion," a scientist studying long COVID told me.

What's hard for patients and their clinicians alike is that health conditions like long COVID exist in the gray areas, along with many other complex chronic health conditions that are not always fully understood. For instance, people diagnosed with lupus may present very similarly to people diagnosed with myalgic encephalomyelitis/chronic fatigue syndrome (ME/CFS), even though one is an autoimmune condition and the other is purportedly caused by a virus. In many cases, people collect diagnoses, as Bethany did, centering one diagnosis as "primary" and explaining the rest of their discombobulated symptoms via other diagnoses. When it comes to these chronic conditions, no two patients are the same. And rarely is there a single silver bullet solution available to *cure* someone. Like Bethany, most people experience a diagnostic odyssey, and this often leads to an even longer treatment journey.[13] This journey often involves a mix of conventional and alternative medical treatments to find a new form of health equilibrium. Part of this journey is seeking care from clinicians who work from different vantage points.

Three types of clinicians typically work with patients with complex chronic conditions. All of these clinicians attend medical school, but their additional training and approaches to treatment and care differ in meaningful ways. First, many people seek care at some point from a physician who practices conventional biomedicine, where diagnostics are critical for health insurance access, although diagnoses are difficult often, due to lack of biological verifiability. Second, many people seek care from physicians of functional medicine—a practice focused on disentangling the root cause of ill-health and that relies on diagnostic tests to identify imbalance, which may or may not be covered by health insurance. Many also seek care at some point from physicians who practice integrative medicine, which focuses on treating the whole person and may combine conventional therapies with alternative therapies like acupuncture, meditation, and massage, which are not covered by all health insurance plans. Many people I spoke to described diagnostic and treatment odysseys that began in conventional medicine and moved toward seeking care from integrative or functional medical doctors in their quests for answers.[14] While some people do go into remission from many of the conditions I discuss in the book, people are rarely *cured* from them. Instead, many learn how to live with their radically transformed selves and set a new pace to their life, often employing a plethora of treatment strategies to boost energy and reduce symptoms.

Most people within these illness communities discover *through time* a new normal and way of being that, for many, brings deep meaning and a reimagined normalcy to their life while managing their chronic illness. This is something the philosopher Elizabeth Barnes has written about: what is *ill*-health, while living with a complex chronic illness or disability, she asks, and what is *good* health, despite living with such a condition? Barnes describes in her work how people can live in good health and have a good life with disability, and can live a difficult life without disability.[15] If we accept that chronic illness is indeed a disability, as many people living with these conditions have advocated for, then recognizing that people may live a good life with an unverifiable chronic illness requires a shift in how medicine perceives the meaning of diagnosis and the projection of care. In these ways, constructing what a good life is and how to achieve it, despite living with an incurable illness, is a social project as opposed to a medical one.

A WATERSHED MOMENT

We live in an unprecedented time. For centuries, people have lived with complex chronic conditions that are unverified and largely unrecognized or unbelieved. The COVID-19 pandemic was the first time in the history of modern medicine when a long-term chronic condition could be directly linked to a new virus that rapidly infected most of the world's population. Nearly everyone was jolted into thinking about this little-understood virus for at least a moment in time. While people were shut in their homes, contending with an "invisible" threat, many people experienced for the first time a deep fear of getting sick and grappled with what illness might do to them and their families. Even in political contexts where people felt that quarantine infringed on their freedoms and civil liberties, people feared the virus and stayed home to protect people they loved.[16] In many ways, COVID-19 shifted how we thought about the world, our own vulnerability, and the roles of viruses in our lives.

The pandemic was also a crucial moment in the history of science and public understanding of what viruses do in the body and of how, in some cases, viruses or their damages can linger for weeks, months, and even years. Initially, people feared the acute infection and possibility of being hospitalized or put on a ventilator. As the years passed, public dread shifted more openly to what happens when the post-viral symptoms stay in the body, although the consequences of the virus slipped almost completely from the minds of many people not suffering from or caring for someone with prolonged post-viral symptoms. While some people recovered after a year or more of suffering from long COVID, others remain so sick that they cannot work or engage in the world as they did before the pandemic, and numerous remain bed-bound. These patients, whose symptoms persist more than three months after an acute bout of COVID-19 infections, are known as long-haulers.

Today millions of people around the world identify as long-haulers.[17] Although, the true numbers are uncertain because there remains no verifiable test and varying definitions and diagnostic criteria. This experience has amplified the isolation that millions of others have navigated over lifetimes of living with a health condition that is unverifiable and, in many ways, unexplainable. Most people disabled from an unverifiable illness must advocate for themselves, feeling abandoned by the state, ignored by clinical medicine, and adrift financially, socially, and emotionally. Monica Guffey, a long-hauler who first introduced me to Bethany, described how "long COVID is a cumulative trauma. In addition to losing our health and ability to support ourselves, we have been disbelieved, gaslit, and not even acknowledged by our leaders that our illness is a significant threat to others. We are experiencing grief and scary symptoms coming in waves that even the best of doctors may not have answers to or be able to help with. Some of us still run into doctors who have never heard of long COVID. That is baffling to me. How are we not educating all physicians about a crisis happening to so many people in America and around the world?"

What's startling about this question is that long COVID is not the mysterious disease it's made out to be, nor is there a lack of understanding of where it comes from or what it does. Instead, long COVID is the latest example of a condition that became chronically pervasive and widely contested, despite our having substantial research on similar conditions. *Long* flu. *Chronic* Lyme disease. *Chronic* fatigue syndrome. *Chronic* pain. These unverifiable health conditions are interpreted with trepidation. In many cases throughout history, such conditions have been considered unreal or imagined, among medical professionals, a cry for help from a hysterical woman. Part of the myths we believe about long COVID, in fact, are rooted in centuries-old misogynies encapsulated in theories of hysteria—an illness category long linked to the womb. These frames were reconstructed with the emergence of chronic fatigue syndrome (CFS)—a disease category that became a cultural symbol of misogyny and medical mistrust. The damage the construction of CFS has done for conditions like long COVID is immense and pervasive, as many clinicians perceive these conditions to be purely psychological despite substantial evidence to the contrary.

Yet, contention around *what* these health conditions are and *how* to diagnose and treat them has cultivated several powerful embodied health movements. An embodied health movement may be understood as patients actively mobilizing to demand recognition for health conditions that are dismissed by conventional medicine in part because they are "unexplained" by current medical knowledge or they have etiological explanations that are often disputed.[18] This was exemplified by the earliest days of AIDS activism, when activists generated an "alternative basis of expertise" so that they could confront myth and bias in medicine to demand health care.[19] The long COVID activist community derived directly from the disability justice movement, which is led by disabled Black, Indigenous, and other people of color who have focused on inclusive epistemologies, centering things like intersectionality, collective well-being, interdependence, and wholeness.[20] These activists were some of the first to recognize that they were not getting better from COVID-19. Many began to organize and draw wisdom and strategies from existing embodied health movements for understanding the condition, sorting through the best strategies to survive it, and drawing attention to the condition in art, medicine, science, and policy.

This was a watershed moment for unverifiable post-viral conditions more broadly, simply because it was a moment in time when public interest put a spotlight on the lives of viruses long after infection, which have for too long been written off. I argue that the long history of symptoms that are defined as "unexplained" or "complex" or "contested" tells us more about medicine than it does about people. These symptoms may be physical—such as pain in the back, extremities, or the base of the neck. They may be psychological—such as dissociation, brain fog, or lack of focus. They may be emotional—such as deep sadness or anxiety. It is important to listen to these complex bundles of symptoms and try to decipher them: not only through the arc of someone's life, but also in a cultural history through which they have emerged, shifted, and transformed. In this book, I track this history, beginning with hysteria and leading us to the present day.

CHRONIC LIVING

Chronic conditions invoke radical transformations to everyday lives. How people adapt to new forms of survival—from sleeping, eating, cooking, bathing, parenting, working, socializing, and celebrating—has been described, according to medical anthropologist Ayo Wahlberg, as new "kinds of living" or "chronic living."[21] Thinking in this way, you might understand chronic living as the ways in which people and their loved ones adapt to living with a chronic illness in their everyday lives, from the most mundane things like eating to more complicated things like transport. Chronic living is not a linear shift, from doing things one way before illness to doing things another way after one becomes ill. Instead, many people who are chronically ill face impairments that are dynamic. People with dynamic disabilities may be able to do something like stand for an hour to cook a meal one day, while they may not be able to complete this task another day.[22] These unanticipated shifts in impairment and abilities are parts of chronic living that involves the chronically ill individual as well as their broader community.

Chronic living is thus never an individual experience. Instead, it becomes habitual in everyday life through tightly woven threads of illness and social relations. These dynamics are not the same between individuals or through time—they ebb and flow as illnesses shift, as needs change, and as people and material resources are available, accessible, and relatable. In this sense, the social relations people weave together through chronic illness involve not only loved ones and carers but also broader communities, organizations, and political movements. These dynamics are all situated within or in relation to health systems—and care-seeking networks. In this way, chronic living moves from individuals and their families to social networks, clinics, and the state in a way that some scholars have described as "continuously contested, negotiated, and in flux."[23]

In the United States, where health care access is immensely stratified due to deeply embedded inequalities and discriminations, chronic living takes on unique (and at times harmful) forms that can produce a kind of liminality where patients endure emotional distress and delayed care and suffer for prolonged periods. I argue that a form of structural silencing occurs when people living with complex chronic health conditions face health care in a culture where complex chronic conditions often remain marginalized within biomedical discourse. In this picture, people are silenced in part because clinicians, who often hold more power and authority in clinical spaces, have limited training in identifying, diagnosing, and treating health conditions that do not have prescribed biomarkers or tests. At the same time, structural silencing involves structural vulnerabilities where people face barriers to health and well-being because of the particular forms of clinician overwork, stress, and rush that have become normalized in American health care when health systems prioritize bottom lines. This stress is amplified when people face bias, within clinical contexts, from medical racism, sexism, ableism, heterosexism, and xenophobia.

This is particularly true in profit-driven health systems like what exists in the United States, where diagnoses drive what tests, medicines, and procedures are bought and sold. When conditions are unverifiable (meaning there is no test to verify that someone is sick with what they think they are sick with), many people struggle with legitimacy, in part due to harmful stigmas that have emerged around some diagnoses.[24] This differs in meaningful ways from what happens when conditions are verifiable through a sign, such as a scaly rash, deep lesion, or biomarker, which may serve to legitimate someone's suffering and create access to medical services.[25]

The problem of verifiability amplifies the challenge of diagnostic uncertainty—a common concern for clinicians caring for people who appear to have complex chronic illnesses like long COVID, ME/CFS, and chronic Lyme disease that remain unverifiable. On the one hand, diagnostic uncertainty lingers when there is not a clear biological sign. Medical anthropologist Abigail Dumes has described how when it comes to diagnosis, "signs trump symptoms," and conditions that present with more *symptoms* than *signs* are perceived to be more psychological in nature as opposed to linked to a biological problem, such as an infection.[26] In some cases, this conundrum reveals serious limitations in medical knowledge. On the other hand, there are times when epistemic disagreements amplify diagnostic uncertainty because there may not be consensus in the medical community about what a complex chronic condition is or how to identify it.[27] In this sense, what conditions are valued and prioritized in medicine are always culturally constructed and temporally situated, driving our understanding of biology, what conditions and questions are considered interesting, how we view our bodies in a particular cultural context, and the technologies that drive our inquiry.[28]

The problem of legitimacy amplifies the need to understand patient knowledge about complex chronic conditions.[29] People spend hours preparing for clinical appointments: leaving work to travel to the clinic, waiting for the doctor, sitting alone in the cold, sterile room while nurses and eventually the doctors funnel through. Many become fed up with language that is unfamiliar and the lack of a diagnosis that drags on for weeks, months, and often years. Most people at some point roll up their sleeves and dive into educating themselves about their health condition so that they might speak more confidently about *what* has completely torn apart their lives and *how* they might find relief and begin to put their lives back together.

Dysautonomia, for example, exemplifies a common health condition that is discussed widely among digital patient groups and that often goes undetected or is delayed in diagnosis within the clinic. I have already introduced the experience of dysautonomia in Bethany's story, although it manifests differently between people. Some people's dysautonomia is characterized by heart palpitations and sensitivity to sound, while in others it may be associated with dizziness and memory inconsistency. Many people experience headaches, migraines, diarrhea, low blood sugar, chest pains, and mood swings. Because such symptoms are common among the complex chronic health conditions I describe in this book, two people diagnosed with different conditions may present more similarly than two others diagnosed with the same condition. This is one of the reasons it becomes so tricky to diagnose clinically.

More than 70 million people globally are estimated to have some form of dysautonomia, and the condition has been reported for centuries. Dysautonomia may develop from genetics, environments, or infections and has been a common symptom of people living with long COVID.[30] Yet, dysautonomia is hard to detect, diagnose, and treat because it often appears in wildly different forms and is shaped by personality quirks, cultural beliefs about health and the bodymind, and social dynamics with family, friends, and work, as well as previous experiences with other health conditions (that may have cleared up or persist). Dysautonomia may also be moderated by structural silencing that is rooted not only in a lack of reliably good health care that people can trust, but also in financial security. Structural silencing persists in part because these topics are rarely introduced in medical school (despite their wide circulation in patient support groups). Conditions like dysautonomia and ME/CFS often receive only brief discussions in medical training, if they are addressed at all.

When patients arrive in the clinic, armed with knowledge from reading scientific articles and extensive social media dialogues on Facebook and Reddit, many are ready to lay out their case on the table. As clinicians living with complex chronic conditions explained, this creates a friction between a patient and clinician in part because they speak different languages.[31] Medical talk, on the one hand, is often confusing, authoritative, and reductionistic, causing patients to shut down and feel dismissed.[32] When patients might not understand their clinicians' terminology or choose to ignore their advice, they can be identified as "bad patients." On the other hand, many patients draw from terms and phrases used frequently in digital communities where people share information about their symptoms, treatments, and clinicians who can help them. In these cases, clinicians who cannot understand what the patient is trying to explain are identified as "bad doctors." This clinical discordance causes patients and clinicians—with the best intentions—to speak across each other, causing both to feel frustrated. As Zeest Khan, an anesthesiologist disabled from long COVID who now blogs and has a podcast, explained, "They can't communicate to each other because they are thinking in different ways."

In this book, I hold two things to be true: that patients may be the most educated people about their health conditions and that many clinicians are doing their best, despite structural limitations, to meet the patients where they are. In some cases, *doing your best* may be punting a patient to a specialist or another colleague who may have a better understanding of the combination of unfamiliar symptoms someone might have. This is an inherently structural problem because rarely are complex chronic health conditions part of the medical curriculum, causing many clinicians to be quite unfamiliar with them. Even so, patients can feel dismissed and beleaguered because they desperately wish for some resolution to their suffering.

There are situations, however, where clinicians cause direct harm to patients. In some cases, providers are perpetuating system-level marginalization—through racism or ableism—which is a common experience of women of color and people living with disabilities, who are often diagnosed later and with more symptoms than women who present as white or able-bodied. In fact, every person living with a complex chronic condition I interviewed described incidents where a physician made them feel harmed at some point. Most also described how other clinicians eventually introduced support in a form of legitimacy and healing.

In what follows, I avoid the terms *contested illness* or *medically unexplained symptoms* unless I am talking about specific research that has described a condition as so (such as in chapter 3 where I discuss the politics of chronic Lyme disease). I find these terms to be derogatory, and many of my colleagues living with complex chronic health conditions find such terms to be misplaced and harmful. By calling the conditions contested, we may further marginalize people who are experiencing very disabling and multilayered symptoms, including those who have been sick for a long time. By putting these conditions into a historical perspective, this book works against these harmful dialogues and attempts to frame complex chronic conditions in a new light.

AN ORIENTATION

I am a medical anthropologist who has spent two decades studying the interplay of trauma and chronic illness around the world, focusing primarily on women living with type 2 diabetes in poor communities. For four years I worked at a large public hospital in Chicago with Mexican immigrant women living with chronic illness. I conducted similar studies with poor urban communities in India, Kenya, and South Africa. Yet rarely were the lingering possibilities of infection, and the crushing fatigue, cognitive disability, numbness, or gut instability a central part of my work. While these symptoms were commonly expressed, they were hidden behind a diagnosis of diabetes, depression, and a legacy of trauma that haunted many women's illness narratives. In fact, in reviewing a story for a colleague about diabetes in Guatemala, I was struck by how fundamentally the patient's symptoms in her story tracked with the post-viral symptoms associated with ME/CFS—a condition that is barely recognizable in rural Guatemala, in part because of a bare-bones health system and limited medical reach. It made me realize that hidden in the shadows of women's stories were profound reproductive distress, nervous and immune system dysregulation, memory inconsistencies, emotional distress, and disabling fatigue that may have told a deeper story, a more fluid and explanatory narrative that I may have overlooked.

I came to this book project somewhat indirectly. Just after New Year's Eve in 2021, my student, Ken Kaplan, became extremely ill from an acute bout of COVID-19 infection. Ken was my mentee at Georgetown University, where I have worked for more than a decade, and we were making plans for his honors thesis research the following year. In an email, Ken expressed that he thought he was too weak to return to school or even consider writing an honors thesis. I helped him navigate his schedule, delaying his arrival and accommodating his needs. As we discussed dropping the honors thesis, I suggested he begin journaling about his illness experiences. Over the next two years, we worked closely together: not only did Ken complete a fascinating autoethnographic reflection of living with and seeking care for long COVID, but also, when he felt well enough, he conducted an early study of long COVID.[33]

Nearly a year later, I caught COVID-19 for the first time. My cough stayed for a week, but other symptoms lasted for months. These were not utterly disabling symptoms; primarily, I experienced severe anxiety and fatigue that ebbed and flowed (and still periodically appear). I think some people who have COVID-19 experience some form of prolonged minor symptoms, like me, while fewer people experience journeys like those of Ken or Bethany. Nevertheless, COVID-19 has run through most households in America over the past five years. Those who were infected in the first two years appear to remain the sickest.

For this project, I have conducted more than 150 formal interviews, often over Zoom but also in person, with around 130 people, 74 of whom were patients. I met most people through snowball sampling, where I met someone informally, and we agreed to do a formal interview. Then, they'd suggest a few people they knew, and those people directed me to people they knew. Some people reached out to me directly after reading some of my writings, including articles published in *Scientific American,* which were widely circulated on digital patient support group platforms. I reached out to others directly after reading their research. I spoke with some people, like Bethany, several times over the course of two years, exchanging multiple emails, texts, or Facebook messages in between our formal chats. Many people who I spoke to once would follow up with me via email or direct messages to share insights, articles, or new experiences and symptoms that they wanted me to understand. I also interviewed many scientists, academics, policymakers, clinicians, and activists working on challenges related to complex chronic conditions. Many of these experts were also living with a chronic health condition or caring for a loved one who was disabled from one. I was struck by the depth of embodied knowledge in these interviews, so I have centered some of these stories in the book. In some ways, centering personal stories and research of scholars and clinicians living with chronic health conditions is a novel methodology and complex task.

Like most anthropologists, I have spoken with hundreds of people and observed an immeasurable number of conversations off the record. Many of these conversations occurred online, and others were informal chats during long COVID workshops and meetings at National Institutes of Health, National Academies, and academic conferences. In most cases, I attended these meetings exclusively as a participant. However, I was invited to deliver remarks to a private meeting of the National Academies of Sciences, Engineering, and Medicine that focused on utilities of the long COVID diagnosis. I also spoke with loads of people informally after yoga class, in my community pottery studio, in line at the grocery store, at my children's activities, and at my university. I actively sought a larger and more diverse sample of voices by partnering with Vanderbilt University Medical Center (VUMC), which runs multiple online support groups for people living with complex chronic conditions. The support group staff invited some participants individually to speak with me, and if they were interested, the VUMC team put them in touch with me.

By recruiting people from multiple contexts, I was able to ensure some diversity among the people I spoke to: participants were equally divided into low-, middle-, and high-income groups; one-third of my sample were people of color; and although I largely interviewed women, one in seven patients were men, and three people identified as trans. People were engaged in all parts of the health system: I interviewed dozens of doctors and nurses, anthropologists and public health professionals, disability experts, and policymakers. Seventy-five people I interviewed were patients, of varied professions; however, many patients were too sick to work and some were employed part time. Before people became sick, they were dancers, lawyers, doctors, bank tellers, hairdressers, pharmacists, police, pastors, and screen writers.[34]

In this book, I attempt to communicate diverse and complicated stories of people living with complex chronic conditions. In my view, common stories have emerged largely in three sets of characteristics, and it's important to emphasize how different they are in relation to *who* experiences them, *how* they are experienced, and *why* people struggle to be cared for within the pluralistic health care system that we have in the United States. By presenting these common stories, I emphasize the role of intersectionality, a term first coined by legal scholar Kimberleé Crenshaw to describe how multiple forms of identify lead to discrimination and injustice.[35]

These identities differ in important ways. First, a common patient profile of people who present with complex chronic health conditions involves a verifiable health condition among patients with high health literacy and who may be white or privileged in another way. Second, a more marginalized experience may involve people living with nonverifiable illnesses who hold individual perceptions of marginalization with otherwise privileged identities. Finally, a profile very rarely identified with a complex chronic illness, even though these experiences are common and often underrecognized in this group, involves people who experience social inequalities and discrimination from intersectional or nondominant identities while navigating the waters of complex chronic illness. Such experiences have been a focus of my diabetes-related work for several years, as discussed in my books *Syndemic Suffering* and *Rethinking Diabetes*. Most people I spoke to for this book, however, were more likely to have some privileged identities through class, race, ethnicity, or education.

One topic I do not address substantially in this book is the experience of children. Attending to the unique experience of children living with complex chronic illness requires another book with a deeper, more embodied methodology and set of questions. I have found, however, that living with such conditions comes in all shapes and sizes. People might be young or old; Black, brown, or white; bedbound or well enough to work; housed or homeless; depressed or mindful. Indeed, people live with complex chronic conditions in different ways and for varied periods of time.

As I have navigated an extensive body of writing—from blog to memoir, ethnography to theory—I have noticed how health and illness are described in nonlinear terms and on people's own terms. The ways we think, who we live with, and how we move in the world shape what it means to live well in our minds and bodies as much as any virus, bacterial species, trauma, or other insults. The ways in which our nervous, immune, and digestive systems interact when our body-minds are off-kilter and what we perceive to be healthy present a big gaping hole in scientific research. This is particularly important for women as we age, because so many illnesses we experience are invisible, misunderstood, and underrecognized, not only in medical contexts, but also in society. Thus, this book is as much about health as it is about illness. I ask: What is health anyway? How do we define who is healthy, and how do we know when someone is not?

As you move through these stories, I ask you to think about how we might build a broader culture of understanding about what complex chronic conditions are, how people live with them, and how we can better cultivate a culture of care for people who are living with them. The person in front of you in the grocery store who looks exhausted and overwhelmed, holding themself up on the counter as they wait to check out, might be one of those people. It could be the woman doubled over with period cramps, whose hidden endometriosis puts her in bed for days. Or the person in the wheelchair who stands periodically and doesn't look sick. Or the family member who is constantly evading family responsibilities because they are too tired or don't feel well, and everyone calls them a hypochondriac. And it is so many others, where caricatures don't fit. This book offers a conversation about the organic pathology, and deeply troubling pain, that complex chronic conditions create, not only in the bodymind, but also in our families, medicine, and society.

PART ONE

HISTORY

1

HYSTERIA IS AN OLD STORY

|||

LENA'S LIFE CHANGED IN MARCH 2020—and, at least at that time, she didn't think it had anything to do with the pandemic. The woman I call Lena is a performing artist and was at the time in graduate school, literally using her bodymind for eight hours per day for dancing, rehearsing, and performing. When the world shut down and theaters closed, it felt like her bodymind shuttered too. It came on quickly: her pelvis went numb, her skin got flaky, and her hair fell out. She could barely walk. Her eyes blurred, stomach ached, bladder leaked, muscles weakened, and she was in chronic pain. She lost all sexual desire, and her memory became unreliable. As a twenty-eight-year-old white American actress aspiring for a career in England's theater scene, she went into a panic: "Literally my whole body was falling apart, and it all came on at once. I'd never experienced any of these things before. It was so distinctly different from everything I've ever known. And all these very intense physiological changes were very real and concrete."

Lena went to several gynecologists and endocrinologists and was shocked when they told her everything was fine. "Why is my cycle fifty-two days?" she asked in complete disbelief. For years, she had bled every twenty-eight days, and after she went off antidepressants, the bleeding stopped completely before it came back in such a different way. Lena had been taking antidepressants for seven years and spent the past eleven months tapering off them, closely observing her body-mind and finding a new equilibrium. The only explanation Lena could surmise was that she was in withdrawal from a medication in the middle of a pandemic. However, these symptoms were unlike anything she'd heard of or could even imagine. She went on to see twenty specialists and couldn't get a diagnosis.

Lena was frustrated and turned to her own research: she had studied neuroscience, cognition, and traumatic stress in university and felt comfortable diving into medical journals. She unearthed every possibility and discovered that some people who stop taking antidepressants develop small fiber neuropathy—a very large umbrella term for nerve damage in the organs, tissues, and peripheral nerves. Many people feel tingling in the hands and feet—this is also an important symptom for people living with type 2 diabetes. However, Lena didn't have diabetes. In fact, she tested normal for every test she took, and her doctors scratched their heads. When she finally had an idea about what she might have, she reached out to a specialist and asked what she should do. "There are so many false negatives," he told her. "You are running the risk of being diagnosed with functional neurological disorder, and then you will just be stonewalled."

Lena was shocked. Functional neurological disorder, or FND, is one of the most complex conundrums in contemporary medicine, in part because it features sensory and motor impairments for which there is no apparent pathophysiology. FND is often explained to patients as a problem of the brain's "software," rather than "hardware." This is why some suggest FND is a modern phrase for an outdated diagnosis of hysteria. For people like Lena who are convinced that their illness is associated with a pathogen, an FND diagnosis can be infuriating. However, like Lena, many people I spoke to were concerned with an FND diagnosis because it can be so stigmatizing in medicine. Many people fear that if you have *FND* written into your medical chart, then you are destined to be dismissed in medical circles for the rest of your life.

This is a major tension of an FND diagnosis. On one hand, neurologists are trained to reassure patients that their condition should be taken as seriously as any other medical issue. On the other hand, even the most recent international symposium on diagnostic criteria stresses that FND is psychological in nature as opposed to a structural disease process that can be seen, measured, or blotted. In this sense, FND is a classic condition for which symptoms must be managed because there is not a widely accepted biological explanation, test, or treatment. FND, still referred to as "somatoform disorder," or even "conversion disorder," appeared in the third edition of the *Diagnostic and Statistical Manual*, the definitive reference for psychiatric diagnoses (although, it was removed in the fifth and most recent edition). The diagnosis, therefore, dismisses the possibility that a pathogen may be the root cause, ending a search for a possible treatment that is related to infection.

Understanding how neurological theories might help explain contemporary accounts of embodiment, or unexplained physical pain, is the focus of Elizabeth Wilson's book *Psychosomatic: Feminism and the Neurological Body*. Wilson argues, "What's pejorative about the terminology 'functional' is the implication of psychological (hysterical) causality."[1] This topic matters a great deal for people living with complex chronic health conditions like long COVID, in part because, in the case of FND, what causes symptoms like seizures and muscle weakness is unknown. Yet, ample biological research has argued that such symptoms might be attributed to pathogens. Many patients find this information incredibly meaningful because there is an *explanation* for their suffering even if there might not be a *cure*. This contrasts with conditions that have clear diagnostic signs and treatments based on physical pathology, like diabetes.[2]

Many people have described to me how they have worried that doctors might use FND as a catch-all when they don't have a better explanation. Lena worried that if they wrote FND in her medical chart, they'd never get to the bottom of her bodymind's unraveling. The doctor told her, "It's better to bring in questionnaires and advocate for testing for small fiber neuropathy. Don't tell anyone you developed this after going off antidepressants, because they won't take you seriously." Whatever else doctors were saying about FND, Lena, like many other women I interviewed, worried that she'd be cast into a diagnostic garbage can that was attributing her pain to, in essence, just being a woman.

CENTURIES OF HYSTERIAS

Hysteria was long attributed to a wandering uterus. The earliest text blaming women's reproduction for illness was the *Kahun Gynaecological Papyrus*, an Egyptian medical scroll from 1900 BC.[3] Women's wombs were blamed for things like choking, cognitive deficits and the inability to speak, and paralysis.[4] Treatments for women were always nonsurgical: swallowing medicine or rubbing it on the body; fumigating the womb with oils or incense.

Hippocrates, the father of medicine, birthed the concept of hysteria. Translating to "uterus," *hysteria* was used to theorize women's ailments—something that few male doctors of the time understood or studied. In fact, the Greeks often linked women's health and sexuality with madness: emotional volatility, hallucination, dissociative states, tics, convulsions. The obsession with the womb by male scholars has been a central curiosity in part because they perceived it as the source of women's undoing physically and emotionally. Hysteria itself, according to Hippocrates, was a result of a wandering uterus that couldn't adjust to societal expectation and therefore was the source of women's social discontent.[5] This idea of the wandering uterus held throughout the Middle Ages and was one reason men were not commonly perceived as hysteric. The womb was considered a "master switch" of all women's health and disease.[6]

Most somatic complaints women expressed at the time were relegated to "hysteric passions"; "heart and breathing troubles, liver complaints, muscle weakness, and pregnancy complications to dizziness, weeping, laughing, absurd speech, and even eye rolling had been lumped together with the customary chokings, fainting, convulsions and contortions in the diagnostic behemoth that was hysteria."[7] This medical framing conceived women as weak, sensitive, and impressionable to control them. When women acted out, they were considered anxious and easily distressed; when they expressed any physical complaint, it was attributed to an emotional liability. These myths were juxtaposed to the "rational" men who exhibited reason and strength that enabled them to protect their physical bodies and minds from life's more emotional events.[8]

The hysteria diagnosis has long been attributed to covering up biological problems in women's health. For instance, Thomas Willis—a physician in Oxfordshire during the English Civil Wars (1642) who coined the term *neurology*—began thinking about what symptoms of hysteria could be mapped in the brain. Through the course of his research—mostly through autopsy—he discovered that in fact symptoms like "convulsive passions" or "fits" may be closely linked to inflammation of the brain. One patient, for instance, died from what appears by description to have been encephalitis. Although little was known about what this swelling of the brain might have been in the 1600s, today we know that encephalitis can be triggered by viruses, bacterial infections, or an immune reaction.[9] What Willis did contribute to the study of hysteria, however, was a severing of the connection between hysteria and the uterus.[10]

Misfiring of the nervous system has long been a focus of medicine, although much of the focus has been on the motor side of the nervous system. For instance, paralysis of the foot, facial neuralgias, loss of vision and voice, tics, deep and disabling physical pain, and chronic muscular contractions were typical symptoms of what was once called "conversion hysteria" and is often referred to now as "functional neurological disorder." Since antiquity, problems with the motor side of the nervous system—from loss of speech (hysterical aphonia) to the inability of eyelids to open or elbows, wrists, or fingers to relax or their tendency to contract, as well as paralyzation of the lower limbs—have been considered physical symptoms driven by psychological problems.[11] These symptoms manifest in many cases in fits or fainting and writhing. These physical symptoms are often perceived to be "pseudoepileptic." For example, many young women with the disabling disease multiple sclerosis were diagnosed with "hysteria" before a biological test was discovered.[12]

Most of these types of hysteria were based on an explosion of empirical research on neurophysiology in the middle of the eighteenth century that transformed how clinicians perceived and diagnosed hysteria. At this point, "physicians would be asking not whether the humors were out of balance but whether the nervous system has become too 'excited' . . . because excited is close to irritable or irritated, they may also ask whether nervous disease was not a result of irritation."[13] It was at this time that thinking of hysteria focused on constructs of inflammation and irritation, and the terms were often used interchangeably—although, *inflammation* was often associated with clear pathological changes at work, and *irritation* was used as a global term for disorder (when the disordered physical site or association was unclear).[14]

During the Victorian era, menstruation and sex became closely intertwined with women's mental and physical health. Many theorized that ovulation was triggered by intercourse and that menstrual blood was a release of nutrients that had been saved up for pregnancy. Most of these theories were based on a minority of patients, and since "they had little understanding of what was 'normal,' the myth that menstruation [was] linked to sex crystallized into medical and cultural lore."[15] Yet, menstruation was rarely studied, and clinicians misunderstood what it was.

By the late 1850s, the ovaries were identified as the true link to menstruation, and illnesses were therefore a reflection of what English physician Edward Tilt called "ovaritis"—often caused by the frequency or infrequency of sex.[16] During this time the lack of sex (as opposed to lack of food, money, or medical care) was often said to be the cause of sickness. In many cases, hysteria was linked to wealth, society, and privilege. In Tilt's view, women's ovaries might become overexcited when women would read, look at pictures, have conversations, listen to music, and socialize.[17] These views were what linked hysteria to the suppression of women's education and power. From this time, new links between ovaries and the nervous system promoted old theories of the link between women's reproductive organs and hysteria.

CARTESIAN DUALISMS

It's important to emphasize here that some patients are very likely living with somatoform disorders, or "real" FND. *Real* in terms of FND translates to the notion that a psychological disorder transforms into a neurological one (with no structural damage in the brain). It's important to emphasize that functional neurological disorder is a medical condition where the mind reveals how deeply entangled it is in/of the bodymind. However, the notion of FND has in some ways become weaponized. The FND diagnosis can allow physicians and, importantly, the family and friends of a sick person to dismiss difficult and painful symptoms that may be treatable. When conditions do have organic pathology, dismissing symptoms as "just hysteria" places blame on the patient not only for their suffering but also for their lack of recovery.

Current popular usages and histories of the term *hysteria* have misconstrued women's illness that can sometimes be attributed to biological origins. Often traced to French neurologist Jean-Martin Charcot, such potted narratives simplify a much more complicated situation. At the famous Salpêtrière Hospital in Paris in the late nineteenth century, Charcot made careful distinctions between those women he classed as hysterics and those suffering from other mental illnesses. The hysterics' symptoms were physical, including involuntary contortions, tremors, tics, paralysis, and what we might now call oversensitive histamine responses. Charcot always believed there were real neurological problems underlying hysterical symptoms—although, he did not know yet what to call them.

But medical times and trends change. Early in his career Charcot viewed hysteria as an organic disease that was measured in what he called "dynamic lesions."[18] Charcot and his fellow doctors were making strides diagnosing things like amyotrophic lateral sclerosis (ALS) and multiple sclerosis, finding physiological causes. Charcot was well known for saying that there is a neurological basis for hysteria, making a distinction between hysteria and schizophrenia that was significantly different from a generation prior.[19]

In the last twenty years of his career, however, Charcot shifted to arguing that hysteria is also psychological or, as he is widely quoted as saying, "Hysteria must be taken for what it is: a psychic disease par excellence."[20] Attributing hysteria to both men and women, Charcot linked male hysteria with traumatic shock, such as from war, which was distinct from female hysteria that was associated with repressed sexual desire or trauma.[21] Later Charcot emphasized how paralysis and tremors, convulsions, and delusions were not faked but rather were somatic manifestations of psychological distress.

This work had a profound influence on Austrian neurologist Sigmund Freud, whose incredible rise of intellectual dominance in psychiatry and promotion of psychoanalysis at the end of the nineteenth century would transform the field. Freud's influence was not only in how people thought about psychiatric illness, but also in how it was treated. After Freud left his training under Charcot in Paris, he returned to Vienna and became famous for arguing that *everything* is repressed trauma. At the time, Charcot's prominence dissipated in the medical community, and Freud's voice became prominent.[22]

Freud believed that in most cases women's pain reflected suppressed trauma expressed symbolically through their bodies. Talking about and through these experiences, he argued, would serve as cathartic release and provide opportunities for healing. Frau Emmy von N was a classic case of hysteria in the landmark book Freud published with his colleague Josef Breuer in 1895.[23] Frau Emmy suffered from chronic stomach pain, depression, insomnia, and hallucination. Freud connected these symptoms to traumatic episodes from her childhood when she was shamed, scared, and isolated. Through an eight-week treatment using primarily hypnosis, Freud argued, he was able to remove the imprint of these "episodes of fright."[24] When some women denied having experienced any trauma, however, Freud perceived them to be in denial and to be test cases for discovering what traumas were hidden within the psyche. Yet, it was later discovered that Freud exaggerated the effects of his treatments—and that none of his subjects were "cured" by his hypnotherapy.[25]

In *American Breakdown* American writer Jennifer Lunden contends that "his pseudoscience still lives, predisposing an entire medical system to distrust women's reports of their own bodily experiences."[26] In this vein, medical historians argue that such interpretations of hysteria tell us more about contemporary culture than they do about the past. Cora Salkovskis, a medical historian who spent years studying archives from asylums in the United Kingdom, found that few clinicians used the diagnosis of hysteria at that time, in part because it was such a broad catch-all diagnosis. This is largely because the idea of diagnostics was significantly different in the eighteenth and nineteenth centuries. In the eighteenth century, the primary diagnostics (at least in psychiatry) were mania and melancholia. These branched out significantly in the nineteenth century, when constructs like hysteria were used in clinical settings to describe behavior as opposed to psychology. However, at the time diagnoses were not perceived to be the rigid systems they are today, when they are traced through illness identities as well as insurance claims. Instead, diagnoses were much more malleable, leaving space for diverse patient experiences.

What's tricky about Lena's experience is that her health deteriorated around a contested topic in American medicine. She never had trouble with menstruation and had taken contraceptive pills for a decade. However, her hormone changes became more drastic. When Lena mentioned this, though, her doctor said, "That's not possible." Now we know that people living with long COVID sometimes present with extraordinary menstrual pain; however, this was unclear in the early pandemic period.[27] Nothing showed up in the testing. There was no clear explanation or diagnostic for her pain. "I was in a position at the time where it was very hard for me to advocate for myself with doctors," Lena explained. "The authority—the power dynamic—made it harder. I didn't know what to say to her." The doctor started backtracking when Lena made a face, saying, "We don't *really* know, but it seems unlikely." Lena was left wondering, "Well, what could it possibly be?"

Today, psychological distress is often dismissed among women. But physical pain is even more frequently minimized or dismissed, especially when it's unclear where it's coming from. This is amplified tenfold for women of color, and particularly Black Americans, who commonly face dismissal of physical pain throughout the medical system. This is reflected not only in the shocking disparities in Black women's morbidity and mortality during childbirth, but also in the consistent dismissal of fatigue, chronic pain, and psychological distress. This has been documented among not only low-income Black women, but also professional Black women, including Black women who are doctors themselves.[28]

Lena eventually found a doctor who would spend time with her, and they finally got to the bottom of her pain. He told her, "There used to be a saying: if you just listen to the person, they'll tell you what's wrong with them. And that when you completely rely on diagnostic testing, you're, of course, going to miss all types of conditions, because we don't have the diagnostics to tell us what's wrong in a significant number of cases." Lena nodded and mulled over his comments, thinking about how time constraints in American medicine make listening so very hard. He went on to affirm her and said, in reference to the other clinicians who dismissed her, "Their dismissal and denial of what you're experiencing doesn't necessarily have anything to do with you, but they're just going along how they've been taught. They're not thinking outside of that framework as to why. Maybe the tools they have aren't working. Not that you're somehow the problem."

It would be more than four years after her symptoms set in when she secured a spot at a long COVID clinic where they explained that it might be possible that the symptoms she experienced in 2020 were in fact related to long COVID. Yet, we will never know for sure. They explained that she may have been at greater risk for long COVID because of the small fiber neuropathy, which has been theorized to be associated with antidepressant withdrawal. Since so little is known about experiences like Lena's, her clinicians wonder if this has affected her fertility. However, her symptoms mimic perimenopause, so it's difficult to know *what* the problem is and *how* to fix it. The problem stems, they explained to her, from HPA axis dysfunction, which can lead to the body's stress response becoming wacky and can cause her body to release excessive cortisol. Lena said, referring to how limited research has been conducted on cases like hers, "Neurological issues are incredibly complex. There could be things happening in the brain as well as the autonomic nervous system in an incredibly complex loop that even people who study neuroscience are just feeling like they're beginning to sort of understand. But that unknowing, that kind of willingness to humble yourself before science, does not translate into the actual practice of medicine."

AN AMERICAN KIND OF STRESS

As hysteria began to fall out of fashion, a new frame took its place: neurasthenia. In 1869, a thirty-year-old neurologist from New York popularized the condition. George Miller Beard published an article in *The Boston Medical and Surgical Journal* entitled "Neurasthenia, or Nervous Exhaustion" where he described the condition as "want of nervous force."[29] Originally Beard defined neurasthenia as a medical condition with mostly somatic symptoms, such as profound fatigability, indigestion, headaches, paralysis, insomnia, numbness, nerve pain, rheumatic gout—attributing these conditions to exhaustion of the central nervous system's energy reserves. He described it as "a physical, not a mental state."[30] The neurasthenia diagnosis uniquely provided an opportunity for men to be given a diagnosis that would soon replace hysteria, even though it held the same position in medical conscience. Eleven years later, Beard published a book, *A Practical Treatise on Nervous Exhaustion (Neurasthenia)*, where he expanded the condition to include more physical symptoms as well as psychological ones like anxiety and depression.[31]

These symptoms can be understood in letters between elite patients and their doctors. The American writer Amelia Gere Mason wrote in a letter to her physician, S. Weir Mitchell (Beard's contemporary), how her neurasthenia had "sporadically left her lethargic, insecure, and depressed." Mitchell was a neurologist known for promoting the medical diagnosis of neurasthenia, particularly among white middle- and upper-class Protestants. It was among the elite that Mitchell and others prescribed individual-focused treatments (like art, literature, and nature) alongside the "rest cure" for "nervous women, who as a rule are thin, and lack blood."[32] His focus was not only on radical rest, but also on ensuring women ate and dealt with their nerves. However, neurasthenia, unlike hysteria, was nearly as common in men as it was in women.

In 1881, Beard published *American Nervousness*, where he associated neurasthenia with a radical transformation of society. He was noted to describe neurasthenia as ostensibly linked to the "whirl of the railway, the pelting of telegrams, the strife of business, the hunger for riches, the lust of vulgar minds for coarse and instant pleasures."[33] In 2011, American historian of medicine David Schuster put this framing into context in his book *Neurasthenic Nation*, explaining how "nervous energy supposedly powered the body in much the same way electricity powered light bulbs and machinery and, just as an insufficient supply of electricity might cause bulbs to dim and machinery to malfunction, an insufficient supply of nervous energy might cause minds to dim and bodies to malfunction."[34]

Beard argued that, "while modern nervousness is not peculiar to America, [sic] there are special expressions of this nervousness that are found here only; and the relative quantity of nervousness and nervous diseases that spring out of nervousness, are far greater here than in any other nation in history."[35] He argued that it was not modernizing society that perpetuated neurasthenia, but rather, personal experiences within society.[36] This emotional and physical exhaustion was thought to be followed by an illness that lasted only weeks for some and months or years for others, and this was thought to be something from which people would recover.[37] The condition became so common that the drug company Rexall marketed the "Americanitis Elixir" to treat neurasthenia, with advertisements suggesting "Especially Recommended for Nervous Disorders, Exhaustion, and All Troubles Arising from Americanitis."[38]

In many ways these changes emerged in the midst of capitalist expansion and the beat of the Industrial Revolution where everyone was working around the clock to get ahead.[39] This cultural obsession with progress and productivity played a role in overwork that so often was then associated with fatigue or malaise. Neurasthenia became a cultural phenomenon that permeated the conscience of writers, reformers, advertisers, and religious advocates (as well as physicians and their patients) who constantly interpreted and reinterpreted neurasthenia.[40] For instance, novelist Virginia Woolf conveyed the immense loneliness and frustrations she felt because of the "rest cure" prescribed for her neurasthenia diagnosis and treatment in her novel *Mrs. Dalloway*. At the same time, neurologists like Charcot were internationalizing constructs of neurasthenia, suggesting that gender was a central difference between hysteria (linked primarily to women) and neurasthenia (not uncommonly linked to men).[41]

As Elinor Cleghorn, a British feminist writer, explains, many clinicians at the time described neurasthenia differently among men and women: "Men developed the condition by working too hard, while in women it was usually linked to domestic and family pressures, or the inevitable fallout of studying too hard when they should have been obeying the limits of their biological destiny."[42] For instance, psychiatrist E. H. Van Deusen theorized that neurasthenia reflected social isolation and lack of social connection in everyday life—attributing this experience to farm wives.[43] American neurologist S. Weir Mitchell found something peculiar when he was working as a physician during the Civil War: bullet wounds caused nerve pain in men that presented in a way that resembled hysteria among women. His treatment was to restore the depleted nerves through electric muscle stimulation, and he promoted bed rest, a fat-heavy diet, and massage. After the war, Mitchell also had a "breakdown" and diagnosed himself with neurasthenia. Mitchell's gendered framing reflected his broader views on women: Mitchell found intellectual activities among women to pose a threat to "future womanly usefulness."[44]

When I spoke to Laurence Kirmayer, a famous Canadian transcultural psychiatrist, he suggested that these views haven't radically changed over the course of several decades. Kirmayer said that, even though mind-body dualism is well known and widely critiqued, "biomedical clinicians remain largely unconcerned with the metaphysical 'world-knot' of the mind-body problem."[45] This problem has been long at the heart of medical anthropology. For instance, in the classic 1987 essay "The Mindful Body," Nancy Scheper-Hughes and Margaret Lock posed the question "What is real?" and complicated the false dichotomies of bodies of spirit and matter, mind and body, and real and unreal that have become vital thinking in biomedical practice through time.[46] Kirmayer suggests that these dichotomies persist despite the fact that science is slowly "untangling this knot," with consistent biological revelations that unveil links between the body and behavior. Thinking about the body as a machine that can be brought to the clinic for repairs, Kirmayer argued, obscures the meaning we make in our everyday lives that influence our bodies too. This meaning is often created through social relations, like dynamics with family and friends, encounters at work or school, and even side-eyes or comments on the street or at the market.

DIAGNOSTIC SHIFTS

FND is, in many ways, the new neurasthenia, or hysteria. Some women I spoke to described how difficult it can be for people who have *FND* scribed into their medical charts to get taken seriously in emergency room or specialist visits in the future. This is why patients are so resistant to the FND diagnostic when they have an inkling of a different cause (like a virus or bacterial infection). This fear is spun widely, as patients with FND diagnoses report on digital medial platforms how they are being denied testing, medications, and being taken seriously in clinical settings.

Why is this diagnosis so stigmatizing? Many women diagnosed with "nonorganic" symptoms then go on to find a physiological cause. Identifying a woman's pain and distress with FND stops the clinical search for an organic pathology. Doing so simply suggests that there is no "real" illness and therefore no "real" cure. In this sense, clinicians use the construct of "real" to convey verifiability by tests. This is why so many people like Lena felt so very dismissed—there was no test to verify their suffering.

This is also not a new story. Over several decades other physicians and professors pushed the idea that the mind, body, and social relationships are deeply entangled. A nineteenth-century physician, Thomas King Chambers, for example, argued in the 1860s that there was no diagnostic classification for hysteria and no confirmed diagnostic proof or sign. Chambers conceived of hysteria as a condition that afflicted the heart, lungs, and stomach—organs producing both "pain and pleasure." He argued that listening to patients and considering their symptoms was critical for understanding what ailed them. For instance, symptoms considered hysteric—"from unexplained pain, vomiting, and catalepsy to palpitations, crying fits, and convulsions—often followed some shock, fright, or emotional misery. One of his patients was a seventeen-year-old nursery maid rushed to St. Mary's Hospital in London with muscle pain, leg paralysis, drenching sweats, and a racing heart."[47] When he dug further, he discovered that she had worked since she was twelve, her father had recently died, she found out by accident, and she lost her job due to profound grief. She started having what is now considered anxiety attacks—but Chambers suggested that it wasn't "all in her head." Instead, her physical illness was profoundly affected by her emotional experiences.[48]

The departure between hysteria and neurasthenia was fluid. Neurasthenia was considered by some a "fashionable" disease after World War I.[49] It "propagated like an epidemic."[50] With so many men returning from the wars, carrying battle scars, the term *neurasthenia* provided an alternative frame that was distinct from hysteria. A study conducted at the National Hospital in Queen Square, London, for example, found that close to half of cases (33%–50%) diagnosed as neurasthenia were in men between 1890 and 1930, and that nearly one in ten people discharged from the hospital at that time were diagnosed with neurasthenia.[51] These data demonstrate the extraordinary psychological imprints of war, which would soon be transformed into the diagnosis "shell shock."

During this time women's suffrage movements were building—more women were going to school, writing, and organizing politically. American physician, scientist, and teacher Mary Putnam Jacobi argued, "A distinction is often made, based upon the sex and temper of the patient. If this be a female, and notably selfish, the case is pronounced hysteria. If a man, or thought a woman amiable and unselfish, the case is called neurasthenia."[52] She argued that menstruation had been wildly overpathologized by the male gynecological literature and pushed back.[53] In 1877, Putnam Jacobi published a revolutionary book, *The Question of Rest for Women during Menstruation*, which "demystified punitive theories about female physiology."[54] It was the first book about women's thoughts and feelings about their lives and bodies that shifted how medicine and the public thought about the concept of hysteria.

Early feminists perceived constructs of hysteria to convey how clinicians conceived the body and culture.[55] The controversial feminist literary critic Elaine Showalter argued in *Hystories* that "hysteria has served as a form of expression, a body language for people who otherwise might not be able to speak or even to admit what they feel."[56] She contends that psychological plagues live on but have been "relabeled for a new era" to shine a light on the scourges of the modern age: "a virus, sexual molestation, chemical warfare, satanic conspiracy, infiltration."[57] In *Psychosomatic* Elizabeth Wilson, however, cautions against taking these earlier feminist critiques to heart. She suggests that "for too long the neurosciences have been the target of feminist censure when they could be active, innovative contributors to feminist scholarship" and that "feminist theories have been reluctant to engage with biological data."[58] Stories like Lena's reveal how important it is to reconstruct biological narratives of women's lives into feminist discourse, especially when the overemphasis on the social or cultural might undermine the reality of the physical disease.

A HISTORY OF POST-VIRAL CONDITIONS

There is a long record of associating epidemic infections with chronic physical symptoms, although rarely are these histories put in dialogue with stories of hysteria. The first known "long flu," or flu where a complex array of lingering symptoms was recorded, was called the cough of Perinthus, documented by Hippocrates in a port city in northern Greece. In 412 BC, this was possibly the first recording of influenza, and the persistent symptoms of "impaired night vision, paralysis of limbs" puzzled historians for years.[59] While many perceived these symptoms to be spiritual, Hippocrates was convinced they were physical and set out to classify them as an imbalance of humors (black bile, yellow bile, phlegm, and blood). Five centuries later another Greek physician by the name of Galen built upon this idea, categorizing general temperament on the basis of certain humors: melancholy (black bile), hot-tempered (yellow bile), laid-back (phlegmatic), and hopeful (blood).[60] They may have been profoundly wrong on the fundamentals, lacking thousands of years of medical insights, but their instinct to connect illness and temperament continues to help frame how we should think about medicine and health today.

Over the centuries, historians have speculated that it was flu that devastated armies in harsh conditions, gave rise to famines, and facilitated colonization by decimating local populations who had no immunity. The armies of Rome and Syracuse of Sicily in 212 BC, as well as Charlemagne's troops in the ninth century AD, were all defeated by fever, not the sword. This was the norm before the advent of modern medicine and hygiene practices. In 1557, for instance, as Queen Mary I presided on England's throne, 6 percent of her subjects succumbed to a flu epidemic before the virus traveled across the Atlantic to wreak havoc on Native populations during an already violent period of colonization throughout the Americas.[61]

But it was not until the Victorian era that chronic conditions related to these flus began to capture the attention of fiction, humanities, and science. According to medical historian Lakshmi Krishnan, lingering neurological effects of influenza were idiomatically documented through the nineteenth and twentieth centuries. These nerve-centered frames varied widely, from neuralgia, neurasthenia, neuritis, and nerve exhaustion to constructions of neuropathy like "grippe catalepsy" and "post-grippal numbness." They included psychological disorders that were sometimes linked to fatigue, like "peculiar and profound" depression, and inertia as well as severe cognitive debilities, such as "mania and melancholia," psychoses, "prostration," or other anxieties.[62] Krishnan describes how the widespread chronic affliction earned its own nosology: "influenza nervosa."[63] Mary Putnam Jacobi also wrote about this concept in 1890, calling it "hysterical fever."[64]

While many in England at the time could recall the fatalities of the 1847–48 epidemic, a new virus emerged in Siberia in 1889–90, which became known as influenza nervosa for its lingering neurological impact. The virus wafted across Russia and mainland Europe before arriving in England. The British called it the "Russian Influenza" because of its association with Russian oats and Russian immigrants (usually Jewish)—not unlike how COVID was referred to (by some) as the "China virus" at the outset of the pandemic.[65] Eventually, the immediate mortalities were replaced by long-standing morbidities, by which, Krishnan argues, the "detailed depictions of the nervous sequelae were numerous and bundled across symptoms, systems, and gender."[66] These symptoms included trouble sleeping, numbness in the fingers and toes, memory inconsistency, cognitive debility, impotence, psychosis, and heavy menstrual bleeding.[67] In part, this is why Krishnan and Honigsbaum wrote that nineteenth-century England should be remembered as "a nation of convalescents, too debilitated to work or return to daily routines, plagued with mysterious and erratic symptoms and chronic illness."[68]

This broad neurological frame was mirrored in the so-called Spanish flu, or Great Influenza, during the early twentieth century.[69] Despite the virulence and far-reaching devastation of the 1918 influenza, some scholars suggest that had the pandemic not occurred during World War I, with so many soldiers dying in the trenches, it might have become more than a footnote in history. Historians Howard Phillips and David Killingray suggest that many historians have ignored the pandemic altogether, even though "the pandemic left a long shadow of suffering and illness." Hundreds of thousands of people across the globe who contracted the virus "either died or suffered the effects of diseases that were closely related to influenza such as encephalitis lethargica, and also parkinsonism."[70] Most link these conditions to the central nervous system, following bouts of severe influenza.[71]

Rarely are the long-term debilitating effects of the flu recognized when remembering the pandemic of 1918. From Europe and the United States to South Africa and New Zealand, clinicians reported that patients presented long-term sequelae, such as "loss of muscular energy" and "nervous complications."[72] This pandemic was the first time that broad documentation of these lingering effects took place beyond Western nations. African death rates were higher than in Europe, afflicting 2 to 5 percent of the population.[73] Howard Phillips wrote of South Africa, "The incapacity caused by the flu and its aftereffects seriously affected the country's economy for some time."[74]

In Tanzania, lingering post-flu fatigue, characterized by "mental apathy, depression, subnormal body temperatures and low blood pressure, which could last for weeks or months," cannot be dissociated from what has been called the famine of the corns.[75] The condition prevented many from planting and tending their crop, which led to the "most severe famine recalled in oral histories of the last century" as "the onset of rain was not met by enthusiastic planning, as masses of the population lay ill, many dying."[76] Similar lethargies were documented in New Zealand, afflicting the agricultural sector.

Two decades later, in 1934, there was a cluster outbreak in the Los Angeles County General Hospital that produced numerous patients who reported symptoms much like poliomyelitis.[77] At the time, polio was circulating throughout California, causing flu-like symptoms and long-term muscular weakness and fatigue that has been compared, and often confused, with myalgic encephalomyelitis.[78] Two thousand inpatients and 2,500 outpatients from around Los Angeles city and county were being treated at the public hospital, and after the initial round of infections, 198 hospital employees came down with a neurological illness, which was called "atypical poliomyelitis."[79] This accounted for nearly one in twenty physicians and one in ten nurses.[80] The number of people infected, as well as those who died or were afflicted neurologically, was much higher than those numbers for polio, which made researchers dig into possible causes. Six months later, 55 percent of staff were not back to work.[81] Women were more likely to develop the mysterious condition, in part because they represented a higher percentage of nurses at the time who were disproportionately afflicted. The twenty-one individuals with the longest-lasting symptoms were all women, reporting muscular pain, persistent fatigue, and cognitive changes. Several of these women were given hysterectomies as treatment, premised on the notion that their uteruses had caused these "hysterical" symptoms.[82]

In November 1948, an outbreak of a disease that looked like poliomyelitis took place at a boarding school in Akureyri, a small town in northern Iceland.[83] Nearly 500 people were infected at the school, and more than 1,000 people were infected throughout three surrounding counties. While acute symptoms involved fever and pain in the neck, those with persistent symptoms had muscle weakness, tenderness, and fatigue. This condition was referred to as the "Akureyri disease," which became an early name for myalgic encephalomyelitis.[84] Seven years after the outbreak, thirty-nine people were reexamined: one-quarter of those who experienced severe acute illness perceived themselves to be fully recovered while half the cohort still presented with persistent symptoms like muscle tenderness and neurological signs, including anxiety, fatigue, muscle pain, trouble sleeping, and memory inconsistency.[85] Among those with mild symptoms, half reported muscle tenderness and one in five remained neurologically impaired. Persistent fatigue and exhaustion were the primary symptoms, and those living with the affliction were often identified as having a psychiatric disorder (or hysteria), much like the diagnoses at the hospital in Los Angeles fourteen years before.[86] A similar outbreak and interpretation of the outbreak occurred a year later in Adelaide, Australia.[87] Forty years later, ten patients from Akureyri were reexamined and only two were fully recovered, underscoring the fact that some people may be particularly vulnerable to such conditions.[88]

In 1955, there was another outbreak that would go on to create a profound divergence in medical hypotheses. This time the outbreak was at the Royal Free Hospital in London, where 292 staff were hospitalized with what was eventually identified as myalgic encephalomyelitis but for years was called the "Royal Free disease."[89] However, it was not the case count itself that made this outbreak so important, but rather how these cases were interpreted. Suggesting that the condition might be myalgic encephalomyelitis based on nerve stimulation testing of the muscles, *The Lancet* published an editorial: "Although they do not as yet point to the exact nature of the lesions, they may provide evidence of organic paresis in patients who might otherwise be suspected of hysteria, and in a disease at present so bereft of positive laboratory findings they may be a help in diagnosis in the future."[90] Melvin Ramsay, a consultant infectious disease doctor at the Royal Free Hospital, was equally convinced that the outbreak was the result of a virus, becoming so outspoken in this debate that the public started calling myalgic encephalomyelitis by the colloquial name "Ramsey's disease."[91]

Decades later, McEvedy and Beard reevaluated the outbreak at the Royal Free Hospital and argued that the outbreak was indeed "mass hysteria" or "altered medical perception of the community."[92] These conclusions were based on the observations that more women than men were afflicted by the condition and that there were no biological signs in the patients. They pushed for the condition to be renamed "myalgia nervosa," even as hospital staff, including Melvin Ramsay, continued to contend that the outbreak was caused by a virus, not mass hysteria.[93] Ramsay's evidence-based response convinced some in the medical community that a biological explanation needed to be taken seriously.[94] This controversy opened up Pandora's box, leaving patients with infectious-associated chronic conditions in limbo for decades.

Medicine has transformed radically since Hippocrates. Yet, there remains reticence to embrace the ways in which viral infections fuel long-term neurological and systemic disorders that can radically transform someone's health. The striking parallels between the Spanish flu and post-viral syndromes that have emerged throughout history emphasize how much information we do have, and how history may be our greatest teacher.

2

THE CASE OF CHRONIC FATIGUE

||||||||||||||||||||||||||||||||||||||||||||||||||||||||||||||||||||||||||||||||||||||||||||||||||||||||||||||||||||||||||||||||||||||||||||||||||||||||||||||||||||||||||||||||||||||||

AMIDST THE CONIFEROUS JEFFREY PINES of Nevada, in the middle of winter, the girls' basketball team came down with the flu. It wasn't long until teachers were sick in the three high schools in Incline Village. In a blink, the virus had spread to the broader community surrounding Lake Tahoe, including a local hotel and casino. The outbreak was quick, but the impact of the outbreak on the community would live in infamy—many people suffered for months and years.

It was the disabling fatigue and complicated symptoms that worried two local doctors. It was 1984, and the winter ski season was afoot. Paul Cheney and Daniel Peterson cared for hundreds of elite white patients in their concierge clinic who had come down with an obscure cluster of symptoms that wouldn't clear up. Curious about their patients' persistent symptoms, the doctors decided to test them for Epstein-Barr virus (EBV, what's often associated with mononucleosis); they were shocked by the number of patients with EBV antibodies. One of them was Sandy Schmidt, a forty-two-year-old marathoner who got so sick she had to quit her job as an office manager. She described how running even one mile "put me in bed for a day and a half."[1] Concerned, Cheney and Peterson reported the findings to the Centers for Disease Control, or the CDC.

Two of the CDC's Epidemic Intelligence Service (EIS) officers, named Gary Holmes and Jon Kaplan, were shipped off to investigate. EIS officers are disease detectives, sent around the United States and the world from their Atlanta home base to investigate outbreaks of viruses, bacteria, and other pathogens. However, Holmes and Kaplan were somewhat reticent about this assignment because there was an existing culture of disbelief at the CDC when the biological evidence for an illness was unverifiable. They joked about the outbreak of mono, or what many people call the kissing disease. Some called it a disease of "depressed menopausal women," and others dubbed it yuppie flu.[2] The seriousness of the Lake Tahoe outbreak was tepid at most, in the eyes of Holmes and Kaplan, in part because their superiors had intimated that these symptoms, attributed potentially to chronic mono or what was identified as myalgic encephalomyelitis, or ME, weren't real. Some called it a modern hysteria. Nevertheless, they packed their bags, with plenty of sweaters and ski gear, to investigate the outbreak located in a ski resort town in the middle of winter.

This story describes the antecedents of how chronic fatigue syndrome was born. Hillary Johnson, in her hotly debated book *Osler's Web*, argued that the snafus created next by the CDC were based on inexperience, skepticism, and scientific missteps.[3] On the one hand, these missteps were based on the recruitment of patients to participate in a study about the affected patients in Incline Village. Holmes and Kaplan started sorting people to classify them within a more unified framework to investigate the outbreak; however, their methods were more exclusive than inclusive. They began by first categorizing patients by their tiredness, and second, they excluded patients who had abnormalities, such as problems of the heart, bowels, thyroid, lungs, muscles, or "similar diseases that might have explained their fatigue."[4] This culminated in a group of ten to fifteen middle-aged white women who fit the case definition constructed by these investigators.[5]

Cheney and Petersen were skeptical of these narrow recruitment methods, considering these "comorbidities" to be part of the syndrome itself. They urged the EIS officers to interview more patients and dig deeper to understand the clinical profiles of the hundreds of patients they treated. They voiced concerns about the methods the EIS employed, suggesting that they interview more patients and recognize that there was likely a viral basis to the outbreak, regardless of whether EBV was the primary cause.[6]

In 1987, the CDC convened a working group to discuss this research and reach consensus on the clinical features of what they called "chronic fatigue syndrome," a condition that has become known as CFS or chronic fatigue of undetermined cause.[7] Without a clear etiology, the working group explained that they chose a more "neutral and inclusive" name to describe women's symptoms from the outbreak, even while noting that *ME* was the common term used around the world since an outbreak at the Royal Free Hospital in London in 1955.[8] Holmes and Kaplan wrote early on that what they were seeing was chronic Epstein Barr virus syndrome.[9] However, they could never conclusively link or explain the association of EBV with fatigue. Cheney and Petersen had a hunch it was something more. "Chronic fatigue syndrome," or "CFS," would soon become the broader catch-all psychiatric nosology, which was constructed by that team of clinicians from the CDC.[10] This is a wholly American construct, which has been exported internationally.

The new label outraged patients. They sent hundreds of public comments to the committee, both in person and electronically.[11] Advocacy organizations for people living with myalgic encephalomyelitis found that 85 to 92 percent of people living with the condition wanted the new name changed from "chronic fatigue syndrome," arguing that it

trivialized the condition and stigmatized them, making people, including physicians, more likely to dismiss their symptoms or ask whether
the illness was "real."[12] These patient concerns emphasized the fact that
such naming overlooked the growing body of evidence around the
viral origins of not only symptoms of chronic fatigue, but also symptoms of memory problems, dizziness, muscle pain, ringing in the ear,
and so on.

Some patients reported that clinicians made comments like "I feel
tired all the time too."[13] Johnson, who was not only a journalist but also
a patient, has argued that the CFS construct erases the contagious factor in the disease (shifting the focus to "yuppy burnout") and dimin-
ishes the severity of the condition.[14] Another patient commented, "I
believe the words 'Chronic Fatigue' are the kiss of death. Who in this
over-wrought, stress-driven society isn't 'fatigued' a good deal of the
time? What people don't get is that this fatigue for people like me keeps
me in bed for days at a time and prevents me from doing everyday
errands and even simple house tasks on some days."[15] Yet, the name
stuck—causing decades of political and medical discord.

The trivialization of symptoms is what angers many patient groups.
To reach some peace between dissenting patients and determined physicians, the official nosology for the condition has been coined as "ME/
CFS"—capturing both terminologies across symptoms and severities
over time and between people.[16] For instance, many people struggle to
sleep, staying awake all night due to anxiety, restless legs, or numbness.
Others struggle with short- or long-term memory, with variance in
what types of memory and confusion people experience. While some
may present with a form of dementia, others struggle with word recall.
Many people feel pain in their joints and muscles and experience
migraines or constant headaches. Others, still, experience night sweats.
While some people experience depression, many patients argue that
their depression can be attributed to losing a central part of one's identity due to illness.

It was possibly the patient concerns that encouraged Anthony Komaroff, who had been involved in the CDC working group, to engage in a revisionist history of the Incline Village case study. He worked with many others, including Paul Cheney—the original clinician who questioned the EIS officers' methods. They investigated what happened to those original 259 patients who became sick in the Incline Village outbreak. The research team collected detailed medical histories, physical exams, blood tests, and magnetic resonance imaging (MRI) from these original patients and found that nearly one in three of the original cohort infected had become bedridden or shut-ins. They concluded that the outbreak couldn't be attributed to a simple EBV infection and that a "chronic, immunologically mediated inflammatory process of the central nervous system" was possibly caused by an infectious agent that also reactivated the EBV/herpes virus.[17]

At the same time, Komaroff collaborated with medical anthropologist Norma Ware to recruit patients with similar symptoms in Boston. Ware was one of the first anthropologists to conduct an in-depth study of what it is like to *live with* such a condition: one of her main conclusions was that the CFS diagnosis inherently delegitimized patient experiences.[18] Most patients told her that this was because clinicians dismissed them because their condition was unverifiable.[19]

Years later Anthony Komaroff was noted for saying, "I think that was a big mistake because the name [chronic fatigue syndrome], in my opinion, and the opinion of a lot of people, it both trivializes and stigmatizes the illness. It makes it seem unimportant, maybe not even real."[20]

AN ANTHROPOLOGICAL INFLUENCE

I came to understand how deeply entangled the CFS story was with anthropology when I began digging into side comments and queries from academics, practitioners, and patients I spoke to. I was struck by various influences of anthropology and anthropologists in the shaping of this nosology. These conversations were framed particularly by anthropologists such as Arthur Kleinman and Norma Ware, who participated in a special symposium of cross-disciplinary dialogue about CFS in the United Kingdom in the early 1990s (which I'll get to in the next section). These conversations took place as psychiatric diagnoses were shifting more broadly, where nosology was very much in motion, and psychiatry itself was struggling to ground itself as "real" medicine.[21] Given the significance of these challenges and the millions of people diagnosed with CFS, I've been struck by the lack of attention these issues have been given over the past several decades in anthropology. In anthropology, CFS has been largely conveyed as an idiom of distress, or a cultural way of expressing emotional distress that may or may not directly correspond with specific symptoms.[22]

I begin with Arthur Kleinman's research on neurasthenia, which originated in Taiwan and China. Kleinman is an influential theorist of medical and psychological anthropology as well as a practicing psychiatrist. He's written foundational books and articles in anthropology and cared for thousands of patients, mostly in the United States, China, and Taiwan. Much of this work was done in partnership with his late wife, anthropologist Joan Kleinman, and she was credited in some of those publications. When I write about this work, I will be referring to their collective work as well as Arthur Kleinman's sole-authored publications on neurasthenia in China. This anthropological work is famously recognized for how it changed the way he thought about health and disease as a clinician because he found that patients told moral stories that had both deeply personal and culturally relevant meanings when they spoke of their illness experiences. This differed from clinical narratives—and their stories of neurasthenia diverged in meaningful ways from what he originally thought they presented with: depression.

Kleinman conducted his landmark anthropological study on neurasthenia, or *shenjing shuairuo,* in the wake of the brutal political turmoil that consumed the Cultural Revolution in China from 1966 to 1976. During this time, Mao Zedong attacked the Chinese Communist Party along with the institutional structure of Chinese society, causing millions of people to be affected by political criticism, physical assault, suicide, and murder. This caused a "lost generation" of young people who were sent from urban centers to remote areas to work, causing distrust, bitterness, and disillusion. Others were imprisoned, and factions emerged within families, institutions, and systems throughout the government and society. As Kleinman put it, "parents were attacked by children; teachers were assaulted by students; Red Guards—adolescent and young adult revolutionaries—broke into homes, looted their contents, beat their occupants, and destroyed precious objects such as ancestral tablets, heirlooms, and books."[23]

For years people felt isolated and oppressed by the government. In the late 1970s, however, the state allowed expression of public loss and anger—this was stopped when these expressions began to influence a public movement toward democratization. In this way, the "social memory of the Cultural Revolution was silenced or reworked in an authorized version, a 'public transcript' that located blame" among some and not others—deflecting guilt of the Party. The "delegitimation crisis" soon reached epidemic proportions that then intensified, as economic reforms of the 1980s caused more austerity and suffering within families.[24]

During this decade, Arthur and Joan Kleinman dually conducted ethnographic work in Hunan—a south central part of the China mainland—primarily focusing on narratives of illness experience.[25] They found that patients expressed bodily complaints to talk about the stress and trauma of the Cultural Revolution period.[26] In his book *Rethinking Psychiatry*, Arthur Kleinman describes an encounter with "Mrs. Lin," a schoolteacher in her late twenties.[27] They met in a sweaty clinical room in mid-August, where she described experiencing chronic headaches, dizziness, tiredness, fatigue, weakness, and a ringing in her ears for years. Mrs. Lin indicated that these physical symptoms had intensified over the past eighteen months. When Kleinman asked if she'd experienced any depression, her face dropped, and she described several difficult things in her life. As intellectuals, her parents were abused by the Red Guards and eventually died in the Cultural Revolution. During this time, she went without food, struggled emotionally, and lived in difficult circumstances. Once she moved back home, she struggled to achieve academically and was forced into an unhappy and abusive marriage. A year before, she'd had a stillbirth and felt blamed for the child's death. She described feeling hopeless and helpless and had fleetingly considered suicide.[28]

Kleinman believed she had a classic case of depression in American contexts. But Mrs. Lin was adamant that her chief problem was *shenjing shuairuo*. Her Chinese psychiatrists agreed that her depression was a manifestation of neurasthenia.[29]

The Kleinmans found at the time that people conveyed bodily memory, personal stories, and social histories into their illness stories through three core symptoms: dizziness (or vertigo), exhaustion, and pain.[30] On the one hand, dizziness is a common symptom of neurasthenia and other complex chronic conditions of the West. However, Joan and Arthur Kleinman argued that it takes on salience in Chinese medical tradition where balance and harmony are fundamental and expressive of health. For instance, while *shen* conveys vitality and one's ability to form ideas and a personality to live life, *jing* conveys the channels through which *qi* (vital energy) and *xue* (blood) travel through the body. Together, *shenjing* means "nerves" or "nervous system." Combining *shuai* (degeneration) with *ruo* (weakness), *shenjing shuairuo* conveys nerve weakness, and together the psychiatric symptoms and somatic complaints closely resemble those in neurasthenia.[31] In this context, to be dizzy was to be unbalanced or to experience malaise and dis-ease. Yet, dizziness was also associated with falling from higher to lower social status.

In *Writing at the Margin*, Kleinman argued that combined together, "vitality, efficiency, power" reflect a "force of life" that animates people in the body and their social lives. Yet, he argues that this vitality is not recognized within biomedicine because biomedicine is so focused on the material body, where there is a view that "things are simply things: mechanisms that can be taken apart and put back together."[32] Focusing on fixing what's wrong in the body obfuscates the "vital essentialism" of human life that becomes maligned with complex chronic illness. In this sense, with vitalism at its core, biomedicine fails to fully capture the human dynamic of illness. He suggests that "there is no magic" in medicine and "no living principle that can be energized or creatively balanced." Thus, such a "devitalized imagery also negates the therapeutic powers within patients, denying efficiency to lay experiences of regaining force and overcoming fatigue. About power, an ordinary human experience, biomedicine is silent."[33]

The second symptom mentioned in illness stories—exhaustion or fatigue—was related to sleeplessness and the weakness associated with it, which was linked to shared trauma from the Cultural Revolution period. During this time vital sources of renewal were exhausted, and personal and collective efficacy were drained. Moreover, fatigue and weakness in Chinese medical theory convey loss or blockage in the flow of vital energy, or *qi*. The loss of vitality was therefore central to social connections as well as a connection with the body-self.[34]

The third core symptom mentioned in illness stories, pain through headaches, backaches, and cramps, conveyed the "effects of the Cultural Revolution's turmoil on human lives." This metaphor was not only personal—in terms of muscles, bones, nerves, and blood—but also social, in terms of conflict at work and in the family. People described how relations were poisoned, aspirations for a good life were put on hold, and interpersonal conflicts and bitterness festered. "The exhausted painful, vertiginous body," they conveyed, "became the grounds of negations over jobs, time responsibilities, and resources."[35]

The Kleinmans argued that people experienced and expressed this pain in a way to embody the moral turmoil they felt in a society that had radically and violently transformed, cultivating a new social order that they found rife with adversity and painful memory.

The Kleinmans link these narratives to stories of Holocaust survivors that summon a link to traumatic and somatic experience. Lawrence Langer described how "deep memory" is a basic core of experienced memory—such as hunger—that persists within the subconscious and continues as living testimony. With these links, people survive within a context of "permanently disrupted suspension" through which deep memory connects that extraordinary trauma of the past with an attempt to cultivate a new normal.[36] Langer's interlocutor expressed, "You sort of don't feel at home in this world anymore, because this experience—you can live with it, it's like constant pain: you never forget, you never get rid of it, but you learn to live with it."[37]

Yet, as Sing Lee argues, the prominence of *shenjing shuairuo* in the wake of the Cultural Revolution may also have been its downfall.[38] As both Michel Foucault and Allan Young have suggested, psychiatric diseases are not static measurable things; rather, they are made-up constellations of symptoms that are linked to time, politics, place, and social practice.[39] One doctor said, "The kind of neurasthenic patients that I routinely encountered in the 1960s–70s, who presented with mental excitability, difficulty in thinking and weakness, are rarely seen now a days."[40] This has been attributed in part to Kleinman's in-depth study of *shenjing shuairuo*, which shaped the local understanding of this nonpsychotic disorder at a time when neurasthenia itself had all but disappeared from American psychiatry.[41]

Specifically, Kleinman's study of one hundred neurasthenic patients in an outpatient psychiatry clinic in Hunan Medical College showed that most patients could be rediagnosed as depressed, according to the North American diagnostic criteria outlined in the *Diagnostic and Statistical Manual*, third edition (DSM-III). However, many of these patients did not respond fully to antidepressant medication, and their chief somatic complaints only subsided when they resolved major work and family problems, causing Kleinman to surmise that *shenjing shuairuo* may be a cultural-bound illness with an underlying depressive affect.[42] Hence, Kleinman originally theorized that neurasthenia was not a viable psychiatric category and shifted his thinking to perceive *shenjing shuairuo* as an important Chinese disease category because it was popular among health professionals and substantiated a strong biological basis.[43]

Kleinman told me, however, "My argument that I made was totally misinterpreted by my Chinese colleagues. Mine was a medical anthropological argument that neurasthenia was an idiom of distress, not only for patients but for professionals, for whom it was a legitimized category. That depression and anxiety were new—since the Chinese medical system had been cut off from the West for 40 years, they with the rest of the world really, in some ways, were in a state of shock about how to engage with the more psychological and psychiatric orientation in biomedicine. And so, they really didn't know how to take this into account easily at the same time. The question that I raised was not only just a question of what is neurasthenia, but also a question of what is depression?" In this way, Kleinman blurs the idea of overly categorizing psychiatric conditions, particularly when contexts of vitality are fundamental in Chinese medicine, while the notion of vitality is largely absent from Western biomedicine as well as from popular belief of dis-ease.[44]

Lee suggests that when neurasthenia disappeared from the DSM-III in American psychiatry (due to being considered too vague and all-encompassing), it was replaced with an overbearing introduction of depression and its treatments. The DSM schema was organized to characterize every conceivable mental condition as a disease to serve private medical insurance and government programs in the United States that authorized remuneration to practitioners.[45] With antidepressants serving as an effective treatment for most patients diagnosed with *shenjing shuairuo*, the depression diagnosis started to become more fashionable in urban Chinese psychiatric clinics and profitable to global markets. Indeed, historians and anthropologists have demonstrated widely that when a new category emerges, people gravitate toward it. Some Chinese psychiatrists—influenced in part by Kleinman's prominence and influence—pushed to retain *shenjing shuairuo* as a diagnostic tool. Yet, this was negated repeatedly in Western psychiatry, which moved, in part through the work of the DSM and American pharmaceutical industry, to link pharmacological treatments to diagnoses.[46] With the heterogeneity of *shenjing shuairuo* etiology and symptoms, depression emerged as a more dominant diagnosis in Chinese psychiatry because psychopharmaceuticals provided a clear treatment pathway.[47]

THE CIBA FOUNDATION SYMPOSIUM

Kleinman wrapped up his work in China around the same time the controversies around the CDC working group on CFS were occurring in the United States. In 1991, the Ciba Foundation hosted a symposium focused on chronic fatigue syndrome, bringing together clinicians from internal medicine and psychiatry, with immunologists, virologists, and social scientists, to "explore the forms, sources, and consequences of this illness."[48] The Ciba Foundation is an international scientific and educational charity founded in 1947 by the Swiss chemical and pharmaceutical company CIBA Limited, operating in London. The Ciba Foundation convenes a plethora of scientists involved in medical, biological, and chemical issues in London to discuss and debate current topics.

The Ciba Foundation symposium was intended to grapple with challenges around biological unverifiability, chronic fatigue, chronic pain, depression, physical manifestations of the disease, and patient experience. Kleinman served as one of two "chairmen" for a discussion of CFS at the Ciba Foundation symposium, alongside Stephen Straus, a National Institutes of Health (NIH) clinician-researcher. Kleinman explained to me that "the fulcrum of concern" for this meeting was focused on whether conditions characterized by chronic pain and chronic fatigue had biological origins, referring to them as "not just psychiatric conditions but also mental health conditions in a broad sense." In the culminating report, Kleinman and Straus drafted an introduction that included the following observation: "The surprise of the symposium was the breadth and openness of dialogue" where the "anthropological perspective" was "defined for a biomedical audience" and "incorporated immediately into the ensuing discussion."[49]

Kleinman's anthropological research in China was a frequent discussion point in the symposium, resulting in a common thread of psychologizing the condition. This was in part because of a lack of biological verifiability for the condition; however, there were many points in the discussion where CFS was compared to several psychological categories, including the cultural idiom *shenjing shuairuo* from China. While many American clinicians align this diagnosis with chronic fatigue syndrome, some have argued that chronic fatigue syndrome differs from *shenjing shuairuo* in part because it is linked to more physical symptoms and reduced social functioning.[50] Similar arguments may be made to other cultural idioms of distress in France (*les états nerveaux*) and Germany (*nervosität*) as well as Latin America (*nervios*), India (*dhat* syndrome), Korea (*hwa byung*), Eastern Asian communities (Khyal attacks and wind-related illnesses), and Mongolia (*yadargaa*).[51] Kleinman and Straus wrote that, as in Chinese societies, where "complaints of chronic fatigue are frequent in patients diagnosed with neurasthenia," in the United States, "such problems are given labels depression, panic anxiety, sleep disorder, and chronic fatigue syndrome."[52]

Kleinman and Straus contended that "cross-cultural differences should not detract from the contribution of biology; rather they should be taken as evidence of the importance of interactions between cultural patterns, social situations and physiological processes."[53] In his essay submitted to the Ciba Foundation symposium for discussion, Edward Shorter argued that a distinction between neurasthenia and CFS—as they were understood in Western cultures—was that neurasthenia was a more all-encompassing category when CFS focused primarily on fatigue.[54] Now, certainly this argument may have been based on the research from Incline Village, which I have already explained was problematic. Yet, Shorter was concerned with neurasthenia when it was attributed to people with fatigue who were not obviously depressed, comparing it to (and therefore distinguishing it from) people with ME. Shorter at one time called such idioms a "similar grab-bag term for low grade psychiatric symptoms that could not otherwise be classed as hysterical (no fits) or hypochondriac (no fixed ideas about physical illness)."[55] In short, he argued that many psychiatrists conceive these conditions—with complex bodily symptoms—to be psychological or idiopathic in nature. This likely was influenced by the cultural moment when psychiatric nosologies were changing and inherently used to shape the specialty of psychiatry itself.

While discussing whether CFS is largely a psychological problem, as opposed to a biological one, Kleinman argued, "One thing I notice as an anthropologist is a very deep mind-body split in our discussion. It is as if one must have a 'real' (i.e. physical) reason for having physical complaints. Yet we know that the unemployed had physical complaints, just like those of people in the first month after bereavement. There's a physiology associated with many social conditions. We must be careful about thinking that a condition has to be either mind *or* body; it usually is mind *and* body."[56]

Straus argued, "The problem is our bias in assuming that depression is in some way different from other categories of disease. I think that view is inappropriate." Kleinman responded, "To me, the strongest bias coming out here is a medical bias . . . when you say these people are talking about *tiredness*. The implication is that patients' talk about illness is just not valid, whereas physicians' talk about disease entities is. Patients are giving you their illness experience. What we are doing is to reconstruct that account as a disease. This leaves a certain tension between our different reconstructions: a first-hand yet scientifically suspect patient narrative and a professional legitimized if experience-distant physician's tale."[57] At the same time, Norma Ware, an anthropologist who worked down the hall from Kleinman at Harvard, explained how patients resist a psychiatric diagnosis because, despite the growing acceptance of psychotherapy and medicalization of some health problems, such as alcoholism, mental health conditions remain stigmatized, and such an understanding delegitimizes their suffering.[58] As such, a powerful medical bias toward categorizing fatigue-linked conditions, including CFS, with depression appeared to be somewhat taken for granted in these meetings.[59]

These discussions reveal how the anthropological perspective was central to discussions in this meeting, framing discourse around how people experience CFS and what it means to clinicians and patients alike. However, reviewing the Ciba Foundation report on the symposium, I wondered if perhaps the anthropological perspective might have been misinterpreted by clinicians in the West considering CFS, much as Kleinman's research on neurasthenia was misinterpreted by his Chinese colleagues. The focus on thinking about the lack of verifiability and overemphasis on fatigue as the essential component of what was CFS remains a lingering ghost, a taken-for-granted assumption that it is closely embedded in depression.

Although these discussions occurred in the United Kingdom, I would argue that the relationships developed there, as well as the ideas exchanged, had an impact on the cultural history of ME/CFS in the United States. One good example is the relationship between Kleinman and Stephen Straus. Straus would play a central role in how ME/CFS research agendas were perceived and enacted for several decades after the Ciba Foundation meeting.[60] Even though Straus was trained in biological sciences, his interest in how one might manage persistent symptoms shifted his view on where and how the NIH might best approach CFS. He served as an influential figure in moving CFS research from the National Institute of Allergy and Infectious Disease (NIAID) to the National Institute of Mental Health (NIMH), a move shifting the condition away from the *infection-associated chronic condition* frame and toward a frame of mental illness. Straus and others suggested that this move reflected a concern around an impenetrable lack of understanding around the viruses that caused CFS, motivating instead for a focus on mitigation of symptoms. At the time, NIAID scientists were swept up in the study of HIV—a disease from which people were visibly dying and for which activism was provoking science and innovation. For the time being, CFS was left alone to flounder as a serious scientific subject. Within the same decade, Straus would go on to serve as the first NIH director of the National Center for Complementary and Alternative Medicine.

CONSTRUCTING A DISEASE CLASSIFICATION

In 1994, the CDC published guidelines for diagnosing CFS under the Fukuda criteria.[61] These criteria required that the condition be recognized as a new condition, that disability was not due to ongoing exertion, and that rest or reduction in activities did not alleviate fatigue. They also required at least four of the common symptoms (like memory loss, muscle pain, headaches, and sleep trouble) to be present in patients. What concerned patient advocates the most was that this diagnostic overlooked what many perceived to be a fundamental feature of CFS, post-exertional malaise exacerbation (PEME), and instead associated the condition with a chronic debilitating fatigue.

Nearly a decade later, the Canadian Consensus Criteria developed the strictest (and current) clinical working case definition and coined *myalgic encephalomyelitis/chronic fatigue syndrome*, or ME/CFS, which is today the most used term. These criteria select for a subset of the Fukuda criteria that involves more severely impaired patients, including specifically those with post-exertional malaise and more prolonged illness.[62] These criteria were revised several more times to help clinicians and researchers better identify and diagnose patients, although the core categories in the definition remained unchanged.[63] To this day, the Fukuda criteria are most inclusive (including a vast number of patients with chronic fatigue syndrome), and the International Consensus Criteria are more exclusive (focused on severe ME cases and PEME); most patients prefer the Canadian Consensus Criteria because they identified post-exertional malaise exacerbation as a major contributing symptom.[64]

Some clinicians and scientists, however, prefer the Fukuda criteria, causing contention among clinicians and patients. Some of the contention around the CFS construct in the Fukuda criteria is its association with what has been called clinically "deconditioning" based on what Martin Seligman called "learned helplessness."[65] The term was meant to explain people who believe that they cannot, after several attempts, change a difficult situation, and they then believe they are doomed to fail and stop trying, thereby accepting their fate.[66] Seligman argued that this was a common phenomenon among people who experienced depression, suggesting that cognitive behavioral therapy might be a good way to promote resilience. Given the symptom of PEME, the ME/CFS patients I've interviewed reject the concept of learned helplessness because mild activity can massively diminish functioning in these patients.

I was struck by the writing of some British clinicians preceding the symposium, which described multiple patients with unexplained symptoms, including fatigue, whose biological tests came back normal but who were afflicted by affective disorders like depression.[67] They recommended that these patients could benefit primarily from cognitive behavioral therapy.[68] Such an approach was fostered in part from an idea that conditions like CFS and myalgia produce a "state of 'learned helplessness,' being potent, aversive, and uncontrollable, and may also trigger or exacerbate the mood disorder that is found in many patients."[69] In fact, they suggested that "continuing attribution of all symptoms to a persistent, untreatable 'virus,' continued to increase helplessness, although it preserves self esteem. Avoidant behavior (which is reinforced by the advice currently offered to patients) sustains symptoms, but decreasing activity tolerance and increasing sensitivity to any stimulation."[70] In this way, they argued that patients feared physical activity and needed therapy to change the way they thought about physical activity, thereby rejecting the notion that PEME was a disabling feature of the condition.

During the Ciba Foundation symposium, neuropsychiatrist Simon Wessely argued that it was important to unpack the epidemiological differences between symptom subgroups of CFS patients—with and without depression—so that effective therapies could be developed. He described how, despite the problem that it cannot be verified, the condition is "continuously distributed in the community."[71] This interest in subgroups may have fueled Wessely's work developing new therapies for people living with chronic fatigue syndrome. Wessely's argument was that patients were not "medically sick" but rather out of shape, or deconditioned, from a prolonged period of avoiding activity (due to thinking they were sick).[72] Wessely and colleagues described these conditions as a "general disorder of perception"[73] for which patients needed a cognitive restructuring of their thoughts and avoidance behavior due to a "self-perpetuating cycle of exercise avoidance."[74]

This may be explained in part because, in the 1990s, there was a significant shift from thinking about CFS as a mood disorder to a chronic pain disorder in psychiatry. This argument was described to me as being due to several reasons based on the understanding that within a community sample, the phenomenology of depression and CFS differed in meaningful ways. In a clinical sample, selection bias may occur because people with mood disorders may be more likely encouraged to seek care, causing those individuals observed in clinical spaces with CFS to have more depression. Moreover, neuroendocrinological research of CFS revealed significant differences between CFS and depression, which became one of the few replicated CFS biological findings.[75] There was also a growing understanding among clinicians that antidepressants had limited effect on people with CFS (beyond raising mood). And, finally, when later cognitive behavior therapy (CBT) was shown to be moderately effective in reducing symptoms and disability in CFS, several studies, including randomized controlled trials, showed that this was independent on any effect of CBT on mood. So improving mood disorder was not the reason why CBT remains a moderately effective management strategy for CFS.

THE PACE TRIAL

In 1998, Wessely and Michael Sharpe suggested, in contrast to extreme exercise or extreme rest, "a middle way of gradual, individually tailored activity, planned collaboratively with the patient, starting at an easily tolerable level and increased only at a manageable pace. Rest is not denied but included in a way that is planned and predictable and not solely as a response to symptoms."[76] Patients were encouraged to push through the exhaustion and pain to rebuild their strength, view fatigue as transient, and question the idea that it is completely pathophysiological.[77] This work infuriated patients with post-exertional malaise because they would experience a resurgence of symptoms after a minimal amount of exertion. Indeed, many of the people I interviewed for this book vilified particular psychiatrists for their roles in promulgating such ideas, which some patients argued were harmful and untrue. Yet, these theories would be central in designing what would become known as the "GET/CBT framework."

For a long time, it was a framework that was used by a growing number of physicians in the United Kingdom. However, a large randomized control trial called the PACE Trial—short for pacing, graded activity, and cognitive behaviour therapy: a randomized evaluation—became the definitive study of the GET/CBT framework. In 2005, the PACE Trial began recruiting patients, putting them into differential experimental buckets and eventually enrolling 641 patients diagnosed with CFS.[78] The patients in one bucket would receive standardized medical care, and patients in other buckets would receive standard care plus adaptive pacing therapy, cognitive behavior therapy (CBT), or graded exercise therapy (GET). A major goal of the trial was to motivate patients to "see symptoms as temporary and revisable and not as signs of harm or evidence of fixed disease pathology."[79] The investigators expected to see that patients who received CBT and GET would show improvement, and the papers they published reported that this was indeed the case.

The trial generated widespread interest and excitement. In 2011, a lengthy article in the well-respected medical journal *The Lancet* reported that GET and CBT improved health outcomes for people living with CFS.[80] In 2013, an article in *Psychological Medicine* argued that 22 percent of subjects who received either CBT or GET would recover.[81] The trial suggested ME/CFS could be overcome with graded exercise and talk therapy.

There was immediate and prolonged resistance to the PACE Trial among patient groups, however. One of two patient groups for patients with ME/CFS in the United Kingdom ran a campaign to stop the study before anyone was recruited; the other patient activist group engaged with the principal investigators of the study to encourage inclusion of the treatment arm and the manual arm for "pacing" in the study. Yet, after publication, the pushback intensified, leading to three major reviews of the trial by the publisher, funder, and regulatory body for UK research, finding no problems with the trial. Outside of the patient community, however, few were aware of the controversy.

Some of the patient frustrations were rooted in the ways in which the science was communicated. Jaime Seltzer—#MEAction's scientific director—told me that people were angered by the communication from the Science Media Center (SMC) in particular, an organization located in the United Kingdom that has been long funded by and accused of pushing agendas for big business, such as critiquing people who were "hysterical" about genetically modified organisms, or GMO food. "They repeated this pattern over time with pro–big business masquerading as pro-science over and over again," Seltzer explained. "For a long time, ME/CFS was their primary target. . . . You can't talk about the PACE Trial without looking at the way in which the Science Media Centre framed how it was received."[82]

This outraged ME/CFS activists, who responded in droves, in part because it is commonly accepted within the ME/CFS community that GET can destabilize and demobilize patients for a long, long time. One bout of post-exertional malaise, for instance, was perceived to immobilize someone with severe ME/CFS for days. Activists campaigned for the release of the PACE Trial data to be released for years; eventually a reanalysis based on the original outcomes in the trial protocol was possible.[83] Over forty scientists and dozens of patient organizations responded in an open letter to *The Lancet*, bringing forward serious concerns about the study's data, analysis, and publication and demanding a new and independent analysis of the results.[84]

A REBUKE

The PACE Trial held water for a few years until a full and comprehensive response could be delivered that pushed against the PACE Trial influence as dominant theory around treatment for ME/CFS. It took a few years for the scientific community, motivated by engaging with the patient community, to produce a response. In 2015, significant events occurred that pushed back against the PACE Trial: One was medical. Another was scientific. And there was a collective activist effort.

First, the Institute of Medicine (IOM) published *Beyond Myalgic Encephalomyelitis / Chronic Fatigue Syndrome: Redefining an Illness.*[85] The authors of the report referred to ME/CFS as a "serious, disabling" condition, condemning the "misconception that it is a psychogenic illness or even a figment of patient's imagination."[86] The chair of the IOM committee went a step further to suggest that they came to those conclusions by listening to patients.[87] The panel suggested, based on comments and testimony, as well as examining advocacy websites and the FDA's 2013 *Voice of the Patient* report, that using the term *systemic exertion intolerance disease (SEIM)* to highlight the common feature of postexertional malaise was prudent. In their presentation, they suggested that SEIM demonstrates clearly how GET and CBT may be harmful for some patients, even if they were not harmful for others. These findings and recommendations were circulated in *The New Yorker, The New York Times,* and *The Atlantic.*[88] At the same time, the US National Institutes of Health issued a statement calling for a more focused research agenda on disease mechanisms.[89]

The second major event was spearheaded by David Tuller, a journalist and public health academic at the University of California, Berkeley. He wrote a 15,000-word exposé of the PACE Trial, entitled "Trial by Error: The Troubling Case of the PACE Chronic Fatigue Syndrome Study," on the *Virology Blog*, a site hosted by Columbia University microbiologist Vincent Racaniello.[90] One major critique was that the extended review of the study emphasized "a bizarre paradox" that meant study participants could be both recovered and disabled at the same time for the key variables of physical function and fatigue. Specifically, Tuller wrote: "participants' baseline scores for the two primary outcomes of physical function and fatigue could qualify them simultaneously as disabled enough to get into the trial but already 'recovered' on those indicators—even before any treatment. In fact, 13 percent of the study sample was already 'recovered' on one of these two measures at the start of the study."[91] A second critique involved a possible positive bias among participants because the PACE team published a newsletter midstudy where they included glowing participant testimonials about the interventions and mentioned that NICE (a government entity) endorsed CBT and GET. A third concern was regarding methodology: the PACE team changed their methods for assessing the primary indicators of physical function and fatigue by dramatically lowering the outcome thresholds from those outlined in the protocol. This was related to Tuller's fourth concern: that the scientists based their claims of success primarily on subjective findings. Finally, and possibly most dramatic, Tuller and the cosigners raised an alarm because there were perceived conflicts of interest with the PACE authors, who had long-standing ties to insurers that were not disclosed to trial participants.

Several events followed this exposé in October of 2015. In November, Tuller organized an open letter to the editor in chief of *The Lancet*, Richard Horton. It was signed by the six academic medical researchers Tuller had quoted in his *Virology Blog* investigation, and it urged Horton to organize an independent review of the PACE Trial study. In February of 2016, Tuller published the original letter, with more than forty signers.[92] Separately, but around the same time, patient activists circulated a petition organized with ten thousand signatures demanding a retraction of the original article that distributed the PACE findings.[93]

Tuller never imagined diving into the scientific critique of the PACE Trial. Early in his career, he was an AIDS activist, and he wrote about HIV and AIDS for years as a journalist. During this time, he had not realized how many people were bedbound by CFS. Then, he went to study public health at Berkeley and came to understand the hidden politics around CFS and its therapies. The ethical questions around the trial were possibly the most fascinating to him: how could clinicians encourage patients to go through the GET/CBT treatment program to obtain social benefits when it might make them sicker? Tuller found that what he calls the "PACE Trial scandal" was bound up in apparent conflicts of interest between scientists pushing the PACE Trial findings and potential financial and/or advisory links with insurers.

The actions of these activists had measurable impacts. In August of 2016, a UK tribunal ordered Queen Mary University of London to release raw trial data from the PACE Study, in the process citing the critical letter signed by more than forty experts. These data were sought by Australian patient Alem Matthees in a freedom of information request. Others were then able to analyze these data, and they suggested that there was a problem with the methodology and that the findings had been exaggerated.[94] Tuller's reporting suggests that the reanalysis showed patients who were presumed to get "back to normal" and had met a "strict criterion for recovery" were possibly double counted as both "recovered" and "disabled" for physical function at baseline, skewing the findings.[95] Yet, in a formal review of regulatory concerns of the PACE Trial, the UK Medical Research Council and Health Research Authority of the National Health Service determined that the trial was robust, thereby rejecting the critics.[96] This is one reason The Lancet has not redacted the paper.

The IOM report was helpful in mitigating some of the medical bias against people diagnosed with ME/CFS. Even still, many clinicians described to me the murky waters of navigating symptoms of postexertional malaise exacerbation and what to do to support their patients who have limited paths to recovery. The widespread acceptance of the clinical recommendations that CBT or GET would help overcome chronic fatigue, even when patients experience post-exertional malaise intolerance, is common but also changing and more nuanced. For instance, an internal medicine doctor told me that often trying GET is a way clinicians navigate a patient diagnosis between fibromyalgia and ME/CFS. The doctor suggested that if a patient responds well to the GET/CBT framework, then they may have fibromyalgia. However, if they crash, they may have ME/CFS. Yet, many patients find a suggestion that the GET/CBT framework might be useful to be an immediate red flag, causing them to perceive that clinician as a "bad doctor" because the framework is perceived as another way of saying "It's all in your head."

Yet, most people I spoke to emphasized how critical CBT is for mental health care, especially for those patients who have been living with a disabling chronic illness for years and see no light at the end of the tunnel. At the same time, many patients remain extremely concerned by the GET/CBT framework for ME/CFS and long COVID. Its sullied reputation within patient communities cannot be divorced from the monetization of the intervention or the perceived potential to cause harm.

With a focus on fixing and monetizing what's wrong, we lose the ability to think generously and systemically about what muddy features emerge in the nerves, gut, blood, and tissues that might be at the root of a misfiring memory or numbness in the fingers. While making discrete claims on what's wrong and how to fix it can easily facilitate what needs to be billed and measured, we lose something essential that is so clear to those who are suffering.

3

LYME WARS

||||||||||||||||||||||||||||||||||||||||||||||||||||||||||||||||||||||||||||||||||||||||||||||||||||||||||||||||||||||||||||||||||||||||||||||||||||||||||||||||||||||||||||||

EVAN HAD A TYPICAL CASE of chronic Lyme disease. She was infected when she was eleven while growing up in Martha's Vineyard, Massachusetts. Martha's Vineyard is a hotbed of Lyme disease—the most common vector-borne disease in America today. It's more common than West Nile virus and HIV. Entire neighborhoods and families are afflicted by Lyme disease. In fact, two middle-class suburban patient activist mothers, standing up for themselves and their communities, were the first to alert the government to the symptoms that came to be called Lyme disease, which had been long obscured or ignored by scientists and public health.[1] Colloquially called Montauk knee, Lyme disease cases have skyrocketed not only due to cases being reported more often, but also due to Lyme's being diagnosed more widely.[2] However, Evan never had a positive test. She didn't see a scaly bullseye rash expand over her skin. Instead, she had nausea, headaches, and fatigue so bad she couldn't go to school. "It hits you like a ton of bricks," she told me. "I couldn't read, watch TV. I couldn't draw, paint, or go outside. I couldn't do anything. It took away my childhood."

Lyme disease is caused by a corkscrew-shaped bacterium called a spirochete (known as *Borrelia burgdorferi*) that is largely transmitted by black-legged ticks. Once the ticks attach to their hosts, the bacteria are released from the ticks, moving into the blood and eventually the brain and other organ systems.[3] The *Borrelia burgdorferi* organism formed 100 million years ago and has been affecting humans in different ways for nearly five thousand years.[4] Some argue that Lyme disease plays a role in escalating dementia in the United States, for example.[5] Lyme disease is recognized by a red and sometimes scaly rash (erythema migrans) that looks like a bullseye or solid-colored lesion (the "sign"). People also experience fever, headache, and fatigue, among other symptoms. Some people experience short-term illness only. However, others, who are diagnosed with or assumed to have *chronic Lyme disease*, experience long-term, debilitating illness, including the common symptom of Lyme arthritis.[6] When Evan's chronic symptoms became disabling, her doctors tested for Lyme disease mostly because of where she lived. In her case, geography explained her symptoms rather than a tick, rash, or blood test.

For Evan, it's difficult to pinpoint exactly when and where the infection took place. The spirochete is common in but not exclusive to the northeastern area of the United States. However, acute Lyme disease infection is not contentious. It's the chronic nature of Evan's condition that many clinicians don't believe, diagnose, or treat. In fact, because the geography of where ticks infected with Lyme fester is such a central feature of Lyme disease, some clinicians don't consider a patient for Lyme disease unless they have been in or live within those specific regions.[7] But that wasn't a problem for Evan. Her mom had it too.

In 1994, the CDC agreed that clinicians should use their best judgment based on blood tests, likelihood of exposure, and clinical symptoms together to make a diagnosis of chronic Lyme disease.[8] This is because the condition is so tricky. Not everyone has the typical bulls-eye or solid-color lesions, and the rash may present differently due to a person's complexion. People with darker complexions are often over-looked for having Lyme, particularly children.[9] Others simply feel their clinicians don't take them seriously at all.[10] Most people are eventually diagnosed by means of an antibody test, where the small proteins that fight infection are identified in the blood. But these tests are not always clear, because the antibody test can't reliably distinguish between past or current infections. Some doctors opt to send blood tests to different labs, which focus explicitly on testing for Lyme disease. This can pos-sibly result in disparate results, making the diagnosis even more complicated.

Evan was treated with a full course of antibiotics. However, when you get Lyme, it's rare that you get infected with an isolated bacterium; some people get a cocktail of bacteria and viruses the tick carries, so the antibiotic may work on some things (bacteria) but not others (viruses). Evan began to feel better after the antibiotic infusions—but that's not the case for everyone. These long-course treatments of antibiotics are a point of contention. Some people worry that the antibodies might cause harm to the body if the person is not sick with Lyme (but rather a virus). Others worry that the antibiotic infusions are a ploy to make money by pharmaceutical companies. Some patients are called "Lymies" to sig-nify their consumerist role in a health culture where patients "take responsibility" for their health when the health system fails them.[11] This name is somewhat pejorative because it signifies how common it is for people to take their health into their own hands and to try any-thing in sight that might put out the fire, to calm their illness.

Evan mused, "Doctors have been saying for a long time that Lyme is hard to get and easy to treat. But that's a total lie. Lyme is easy to get and extremely difficult to treat once the disease is allowed to become chronic."

I was struck by Evan's phrase "allowed to become chronic" because I had read about clinical contestations of chronic Lyme disease so frequently in memoir, nonfiction, and scholarly writing. In her Lyme disease memoir *Invisible Kingdom*, writer Megan O'Rourke recalls, "In the middle of the night, when I woke in the dark with my heart pounding, what *really* terrified me was the conviction that my doctors did not believe me, and so I would never have partners in my search for answers—and treatments. How could I get better if no one thought I was sick?"[12]

Anthropologist Joe Dumit was the first to use the phrase "illnesses you have to fight to get" to describe complex chronic conditions that may be contested in medical and social circles.[13] In his extensive work on "emerging, contested illnesses," Dumit defines conditions like chronic Lyme disease by five features. The first feature is that such conditions are inherently chronic and do not fit neatly into discrete disease models for diagnosis or care. The second feature is that the etiology is unclear and the reasons behind the progression of the illness are also unclear. In many cases, clinicians perceive these conditions to be functional, returning to the adage that the condition is "all in your head." Part of this critique is mired in a third feature too because, as Dumit suggests, something that characterizes chronic Lyme disease is that it rarely exists in isolation from other chronic health conditions; rather, in what he describes as "fuzzy boundaries" among diagnoses, health conditions are often overlapping and cross-linked.[14] The common occurrences of dysautonomia, chronic pain, depression and anxiety, and small fiber neuropathy are a good example of this.

The fourth feature involves therapies.[15] Many people describe how not only are diagnoses hard to get, but therapies that alleviate symptoms are also hard to find. This often leads people to seek care from multiple sources, often weaving together medical and nonmedical therapies, such as herbal tinctures, teas, nutritional supplements, and hyperbaric oxygen chambers. This is tricky because Dumit's fifth feature involves the fact that such health conditions become legally explosive because it's difficult to document *what* is causing someone's illness and *why* they can't work and need disability status.[16] For some, seeking disability may further complicate their situation when disability may qualify or disqualify someone from claiming medical insurance and governmental supplementary income. For others, such as in the case of chronic Lyme disease, the condition becomes legally explosive because doctors are divided by what they believe the guidelines for treating these patients should be. They are so divided, in fact, that there are two sets of guidelines that have emerged.

Medical anthropologist Abigail Dumes argues in her powerful book *Divided Bodies: Lyme Disease, Contested Illness, and Evidence Based Medicine* that a sixth feature is this fundamental chasm within the practice of medicine itself. Dumes argues that within clinical medicine, "bodies of *thought* are divided" that fundamentally shape *what* clinicians think Lyme is and *how* patients should be treated. This results in, she contends, "those who live, diagnose, and treat contested illness [and] often make corollary and competing claims" about whether the diseases are real and how clinicians should identify and treat patients.[17]

I found in my research that epistemic disagreements and related diagnostic uncertainty among clinicians influence how clinicians may respond to patients with complex arrays of symptoms. Multiple clinicians suggested that diagnostic uncertainty may cause some clinicians to punt a patient to another colleague through referral, or to identify another diagnosis that can be treated with more confidence. Diagnostic uncertainty also cultivates a difficult illness experience for patients because they struggle to understand not only why they are so sick, but also why treatments cannot address their most troubling symptoms.[18] These (mis)diagnoses can leave people in limbo, struggling to understand why their bodies are unraveling for years.

MOLLY'S STORY

Early on in my research, I reached out to Molly, a childhood friend who had lived with chronic Lyme disease for years. Molly developed Lyme disease when her children were in diapers, and now her eldest twins are thinking about college. We reminisced about our shared passion for medicine when we were young and how our lives had developed in circuitous paths. After she had her twin boys, she left work to raise them and loved it so much she decided to homeschool her five children. However, after her third pregnancy and fourth child, she became so sick she could not care for them. This was a profoundly troubling time for their family.

It all began with a tick. Molly started camping more when she started dating her husband, and it's become a central feature of their family life. She often pulls ticks off her family members' bodies. Yet, Molly is the only one who they know was infected with a long debilitating illness from a tick-borne disease. "My story, Emily, is a long and painful one," she told me while she was launching into a lengthy story about the six years it took her to get a diagnosis. These years were mired in fear, unexplainable pain, and diagnostic uncertainty.

In 2010, Molly suddenly had migraines for the first time. They were random and episodic—she described how she began to have twenty migraines a month. These were not her only symptom: she developed dysautonomia with the telltale signs of muscle weakness, vertigo, and fatigue. She became so sick she was wheelchair bound for six months. It was then when her husband took a leave of absence from his teaching job to care for her. This was no small sacrifice: not only was he the only income earner, but also they were caring for four children under four. They started to wonder what they'd do for money if she never recovered.

Molly was living in a midsize city in the Midwest when she first had a neurological workup. Her doctors thought she had multiple sclerosis, or MS. MS is a disabling disease of the brain and spinal cord that has no cure. For years, people with MS were diagnosed with hysteria. However, that changed when a verifiable test was developed. Usually, neurologists diagnose MS by ruling out other conditions: they take samples from the blood and cerebrospinal fluid to look for biomarkers, abnormal antibodies, or infections. They also use an MRI to look for lesions in the brain or spinal cord, which often confirm an MS diagnosis. There are also electrical signals that can be gathered from probes within the nervous system to observe visual patterns of nerve movement in your legs and arms. All this information is pooled to diagnose someone with MS. Although, these pooled tests indicated that Molly didn't have MS.

This was one of the hardest moments. She knew she didn't have a condition she feared, which was good, but her doctors could not explain her debilitating physical pain. This fear and uncertainty, coupled with her physical discomfort, caused her depression to spiral.

At the same time, the diagnostic uncertainty around Molly's condition unsettled her clinicians. One suggested that possibly her chronic migraines, fatigue, and muscle aches were linked to having four children under the age of four at home. This is common in medicine—where women's fatigue, infections, or autoimmune conditions are perceived by clinicians as hysteria or feminine malaise—and it underscores the ways in which women are distrusted in the most mundane interactions.[19] This is also a common way in which "long-held gender stereotypes" are used to "make sense" of chronic Lyme disease.[20] When women push back, clinicians label them as "bad" patients. Molly was deeply frustrated by how these physicians questioned her authenticity, which fostered extraordinary distrust.

Molly met with nearly every neurologist in the university hospital, but nobody could diagnose her with anything concrete. When I asked her about her nerve pain, she described how the slightest brush of her skin would send shooting pain up her legs. "My legs would just crumble under me, and I wouldn't be able to walk." This was the period when she relied on a wheelchair, although these flares were periodic. The pain was overwhelming—but the stress on the family and burden of living far from family was harder. Not long after this, they moved across the state to live closer to family who could support them.

It was after the move when Molly found a functional medicine doctor who said, "Listen! Have you ever thought you might have Lyme disease?"

She scoffed at first and said, "Everyone I've talked to has said that chronic Lyme disease is not a real disease, so I don't really know what to say."

LYME WARS

The concept of chronic Lyme disease is incredibly divisive among some clinicians. Some clinicians do not recognize that chronic Lyme disease exists at all. Others take it very seriously. In fact, *chronic* Lyme disease is so controversial that many people call these disagreements the "Lyme wars."[21] These Lyme wars are essentially based on ideas about *what* is chronic Lyme disease and *how it* should be treated.[22] There are two competing frameworks that clinicians contend with when thinking about identifying and treating *chronic* Lyme disease.

The first framework is often adopted by mainstream or conventional physicians. This group argues that chronic Lyme disease does not have a biological basis because it lacks verifiability. In these cases, patients would be perceived to have symptoms with a functional origin, meaning there is no biological basis but rather the condition is psychological. As a result, these clinicians may attribute an alternate etiology or diagnosis to explain these symptoms because they might not believe that Lyme disease can be chronic.[23] The second framework involves clinicians who are called "Lyme literate" because they argue that chronic Lyme disease has a biological basis, and they treat patients based on their symptoms, often involving antibiotics and other, non-medical treatments.[24] In general, Lyme-literate physicians are trained in conventional medicine but break off into a practice that could be characterized as functional medicine, or they adopt what is often described as a more integrative approach. This is not without controversy. Some conventional physicians consider integrative or functional physicians to be practicing medicine out of scope, causing disagreements within the hierarchies of clinical medicine.

When I asked Abigail Dumes whether differences in political sensibilities contributed to the Lyme wars, she explained that people on both sides of the political spectrum in the United States can be part of what she called "cultures of treatment seeking" where people regardless of political leanings "are drawn to complementary and alternative medicine." The primary divisions are instead drawn within "epistemic tensions" in medicine, where clinicians think about what the root of chronic persistence of Lyme disease could be, and if what we call *chronic* Lyme disease is associated with the bacteria or something else entirely.[25]

Debates have largely been attributed to what people perceive to be good evidence for Lyme disease.[26] In 2000, the Infectious Diseases Society of America (IDSA), in collaboration with the American Academy of Neurology and the American College of Rheumatology, developed "evidence-based" clinical practice guidelines to prevent, diagnose, and treat Lyme disease. These guidelines were based on four studies that suggested that long-term antibiotic treatment of patients with persistent chronic symptoms were no more effective than placebo.[27] The IDSA guidelines suggest that treating Lyme patients with two weeks of antibiotics (typically doxycycline) should be sufficient to clear up most cases of Lyme disease and the more serious cases might require intravenous antibiotics for up to a month.[28]

Not everyone agreed with the IDSA guidelines. Many clinicians who work closely with chronic Lyme disease patients believe much lengthier treatments of antibiotics are required. These critics argue that IDSA guidelines were generated based on consensus-based, as opposed to evidence-based, methods.[29] This meant that bias was possibly embedded in those guidelines, and therefore they served to provide clinicians with the authority to rule out chronic Lyme disease when there was no other biological sign to pin the symptoms on Lyme.

Many patient organizations sent emails to patients and physicians across the country to inform them of the current political and medical battles that had become so entangled in the chronic Lyme disease debates. Possibly the most vocal response of clinicians was from the International Lyme and Associated Diseases Society, or ILADS, which was formed in 1999 by clinicians working in Lyme-endemic regions, like Connecticut and Massachusetts. This is the only physician-led Lyme organization that formed to fight against medical hegemony that patients perceived was embedded in the IDSA guidelines.

Many of these ILADS clinicians had found that some patients remained quite ill after receiving long-term oral and intravenous antibiotics, which they administered for sometimes months or even years. Highlighting research not considered by the IDSA, including studies that demonstrated bacterial persistence in animals and humans with Lyme disease even after they had been treated, the ILADS clinicians proposed an alternative "standard of care" to the IDSA guidelines. It defined the illness more broadly, recognizing that Lyme infections can leave people sick for years and encouraging a more extensive treatment.[30]

Part of the disagreement here involves what information is considered valuable "evidence." To understand this, we must consider the history and power that evidence-based medicine holds in medical settings, which sociologists Stefan Timmermans and Marc Berg have argued can "reinforce monopolies of knowledge."[31] In this way of thinking, there are randomized controlled trials (RCTs) on the one hand, which are viewed as the most powerful source of medical evidence, and expert opinion on the other, which is viewed as a significant but less powerful source of evidence. In the case of type 2 diabetes, for example, evidence-based medicine relies on RCTs that have worked with large samples to unpack biological and behavioral pathways to improved health. These RCTs are not without substantial critiques but prove to be powerful sources of knowledge about what interventions work to mitigate glucose intolerance, in part because there is a defined problem, clear intervention—often a pharmaceutical—and a measurable biological outcome.[32]

Dumes argues in *Divided Bodies* that evidence-based medicine has functioned, in the case of chronic Lyme disease, in a way somewhat counterintuitive to what was originally intended. She suggests that evidence-based medicine gave a range of stakeholders inside and outside of medicine (including patients) a platform to make claims around what clinical guidelines should be prioritized. This has resulted in escalating contestation instead of reducing it. Further contention arises, Dumes argues, when "the interpretation held by the more powerful entity is the one that is perceived to be more legitimate."[33] It is this problem with power and legitimacy that has ILADS physicians so frustrated with the IDSA guidelines, and what eventually inspired them to create their own clinical guidelines based on another set of studies and clinical observations.

SEEKING SOLUTIONS

Molly didn't return to the conversation about testing for chronic Lyme disease with her new doctor until her pain was so bad that she couldn't walk or move her arms. Her husband had to wash her and care for her like a child. When she was too sick to seek more answers, they admitted her through the emergency room at a large university hospital's neural department, where they started running tests.

It was in the emergency room when Molly asked if they could test her for Lyme disease for the first time. The ER doctor looked at Molly and said there was no Lyme disease in Missouri. He refused to even test her. Instead, he sent her home with a cane and recommended that she try Tai Chi.

Molly returned to her functional medicine doctor and asked him to test her. They sent her test to the IGenX lab in California, a place Molly called the gold standard for chronic Lyme disease testing. While sending the test in the mail, the doctor said to her, "I can test for this, but I can't diagnose you with chronic Lyme because it would put my medical license in jeopardy."

Molly nodded reluctantly and felt devastated until he followed up with, "But I do know a doctor downstate who is just doing Lyme cases. He doesn't accept insurance because if he did, he would lose his license." Soon after Molly had a positive test from the IGenX lab, she went to see the specialist downstate. He began with a massive amount of testing and treatments.

"Some of his treatments helped and others made things worse," Molly said. She saw the clinician downstate for about a year and a half and primarily received antibiotic treatment. Eventually he recommended she stop the treatment because it was too much for her.

Molly switched to a Lyme doctor closer to home who started herbal Lyme therapies. She started following the new protocols and combined this treatment with care from an endocrinologist to balance her thyroid and obstetrician to manage her hormones. She followed a careful diet and took a daily pill to prevent migraines, manage her thyroid, and balance her hormones. To manage these conditions together, she sought care from a functional medicine physician, a neurologist, and an obstetrician. She also does sauna therapy to help with chronic inflammation and takes high levels of vitamins C and D and probiotics. "You have to tackle everything all at once," she said emphatically.

Molly provides a classic thresholds metaphor, referring to a pot of boiling water: "Everything is simmering just below the surface," she explained. "You add this infectious agent to the mix, and the pot boils over. To stop it from boiling, you must rebalance all the factors at play." For Molly, it was low thyroid, low hormones, and eventually the Lyme infection. The infection pushes people over a threshold, activating an unraveling of the heart, mind, liver, thyroid, hormones—and tips a delicate balance. "And so," Molly told me, "in order to get that to stop boiling, you have to bring the heat down. You must address all those factors."

Eventually Molly brought the heat down and her chronic Lyme disease went into remission. For years she lived well, until the global pandemic struck. When Molly got COVID-19, she felt a similar weakening of limbs and fogginess of memory set in after her acute symptoms faded away. However, this time, she was ready. She doubled down on the preventive therapies that she had found worked for her during her Lyme recovery journey, and she found her symptoms stayed only a few months. She was relieved when her strength came back and felt validated by her ability to perceive her bodymind's strengths and weaknesses. However, now Molly faces a new and serious health challenge that was unexpected. She continues to navigate these thresholds with caution and care, embraced by her family.

THE COSTS OF CARE

How people fight to get care is inextricably linked to time and timing—for things that are critical and urgent. Molly, for example, pivoted to seek a Lyme doctor only after she went through a formidable crisis that challenged her life as she knew it. She was wheelchair bound and needing around-the-clock care, while her babies needed her attention. Moving across the country in crisis was a radical move to support her family. However, this move also cultivated an opportunity to shift and seek for a doctor who might find a solution to her illness. I would argue that the backdrop of her suffering was the epistemic tensions around Lyme that reinforced the diagnostic uncertainty that left Molly in limbo for so long. It was at this transitive moment, however, when she—again in a moment of crisis—considered testing for chronic Lyme disease. These moments of crisis force people to peel back the sources of healing within the pluralistic healthcare system of the United States, which is culturally divided and financially unlevel.

Finding a physician who will treat you and a treatment that works to mitigate the effects of chronic Lyme disease is not only difficult but also costly.[34] Some argue that the epistemic tensions between conventional and Lyme-literate physicians may be somewhat tied to hidden features promoted by insurance companies. For instance, many conventional Lyme physicians object to calling the Lyme-literate approach a "standard of care," because it's not based on the IDSA guidelines. Lyme-literate physicians, however, argue their approaches to diagnosing and treating Lyme disease are based on a more holistic body of research than conventional standards.[35] Lyme-literate physicians argue that when you "follow the money," insurance companies hold back payments for Lyme patients because of the high costs of treatment. It appears that the insurance companies prefer the IDSA "standard of care" guidelines because they limit the amount of money that can be spent in finding a solution for each patient.[36] This results in a high cost attributed to Lyme-literate physicians, in part because insurance companies will not pay for lengthier treatment of antibiotic or alternative therapies.

The cost of care for chronic Lyme can be extraordinary, causing some Lyme patients and clinicians to become caught up in court battles, administrative hoops, and even legislative processes for years. These legal situations are critical for sick people, particularly when they do not have a diagnosis, in attaining disability, health insurance, and other crucial services they need to survive their disabling conditions.[37] Many of these court battles are associated with the IDSA guidelines. These guidelines recommend that clinicians stick to a certain amount and length of antibiotic treatment, and they recommend against including a longer dose of antibiotics or alternative therapies. Patients perceive conventional clinicians who adhere to this restriction of treatment to be significant gatekeepers in accessing the medications that Lyme patients perceive they need.

Many patients seek a "therapeutically diverse" collection of conventional and alternative therapies like those Molly described.[38] While many treatments, such as antibiotics and massage, may be covered by health insurance, many other tests and treatments are not covered, because they are considered experimental or peripheral to what is perceived to be "medical" care. These treatment costs serve as a "significant financial barrier to identifying as a chronic Lyme patient or being diagnosed with chronic Lyme disease."[39] It is these financial barriers and burdens that become part of chronic living with Lyme and other complex chronic conditions because the cost of care affects not only the patient but, in some cases, entire families and communities. For instance, many people pay for care through crowdsourcing funds on platforms like GoFundMe.[40] Molly and Evan were both able to cover the financial burdens introduced by living with an unverified complex chronic condition (even at great cost), but not everyone can do so. While such therapies can bring relief, they also introduce an extraordinary chasm between *who can fight to get this care* and who find this care too expensive to consider in the first place.

4

PAIN WITHOUT VERIFIABILITY

|||

PHILOSOPHER SUSAN SONTAG FAMOUSLY CRITIQUED the ways in which American culture uses illness as metaphor—a way to conflate the body as a moral matter where any signal of physical disease is perceived to reflect internal flaws.[1] This is one reason psychological theories of illness can be so harmful: they blame people who are suffering for being sick. This can feel incredibly heavy for people living with complex chronic illnesses, especially as they continue to unpack the layers of trauma that have consumed a life. At the same time, such cultural blame can make the searing pain worse, embodying for some a deep unrelenting shame—particularly when treatments don't fix it.[2]

Most patients who have pain without verifiability are searching for explanations for why they got sick and how to improve their health and well-being so they can function in the world and pursue a meaningful life in the way they imagine. The problem is, there are no simple answers.

Instead, understanding complex chronic illnesses like ME/CFS, chronic Lyme disease, and long COVID is a tricky endeavor. The thresholds metaphor helps us think about how people's sickness emerges and is embodied. It requires us to push back against dominant narratives in medicine that focus on singular diseases and clear-cut pathologies. Instead, thinking in terms of thresholds provides us with a much more holistic story of why people get sick and how people might engage in a path to recovery.

In my mind, thresholds are tipping points that occur when the body-mind cannot sustain a level of health, due to the multiple insults that have diminished its strength. These insults or, as Chinese medicine doctor Brooke Moen called them, "invaders" build on one another through time and begin to unravel and dysregulate the body. These include viruses, bacteria, stress, trauma, fungi, parasites, foods, chemicals, and other things that manage to enter the bodymind through the mouth, skin, and emotions. In some ways, the thresholds metaphor incorporates concepts from epidemiology and biology, such as weathering, allostatic load, and exposomes, that suggest that cumulative burdens over the life course build on one another to cause sickness.[3] People perceive and experience these threats differently, and thus such perceptions and physiological responses can wildly differ and affect people in significant and divergent ways. Mixed and stirred with more material invaders, the bodymind can easily exceed an equilibrium it can easily bounce back to.

Writer and biologist Robert Sapolsky offers a useful metaphor in his popular book on stress and disease, *Why Zebras Don't Get Ulcers*. He states, "Put two little kids on a seesaw, and they can pretty readily balance themselves on it. This is allostatic balance when nothing stressful is going on, with the children representing the low levels of various stress hormones. . . . In contrast, the torrents of those same stress hormones released by a stressor can be thought of as two massive elephants on the seesaw. With great effort, they can balance themselves as well. But if you constantly try to balance a seesaw with two elephants instead of two kids, all sorts of problems emerge."[4] In other words, thresholds are overcome when the stress response puts too much into motion, occupying too much of the bodymind's focus and halting other long-term projects like digestion, growth, reproduction, tissue repair, and immunity. For some, the damage is done simply by the enormity of invaders that wear down the bodymind. For others, when stress has ravaged the bodymind, it's hard for the bodymind to calm down and rest.[5] In all these cases, it can be difficult to pinpoint *exactly* what pushed the body over the threshold.

Let me explain with the story of Tamara Brand, who goes by Tam. This story is an extreme case where the threshold was significantly altered early in life, making the search for stabilization a lifelong journey. Her experiences reveal how cumulative threats that occur over a life course may not always be clear and in many ways may blur together or overlap. These aggregate insults become emboldened in chronic living, when the physical reality of pain in the gut, pelvis, muscles, head, and elsewhere may be silenced in society or medical settings. In what follows, Tam's story reveals the extraordinary impact of unverifiable illness and chronic pain that has caused her to become an expert on her health condition, in part because it is so foreign to every clinician she has ever encountered.

TAM'S STORY

Tam's childhood was messy. She grew up as a latchkey kid in a white family in rural Minnesota scrambling to get by in the eighties. Tam's parents worked hard, but family life was up-and-down. The first time she landed in the emergency room was when she was fifteen. Tam's pelvic area and lower back were cramping in pain so intense, it felt like someone was stabbing her repeatedly. She would get dizzy and nauseated when she tried to stand. She'd throw up, double over, and fall into a puddle of tears from the pain. When she talks about her childhood, Tam often describes the "medical gaze" of clinicians who didn't take her pain seriously, often dismissing her.[6] The only one who did believe her was her mom. Tam was eventually diagnosed with endometriosis (a diagnosis her mother had too). She popped Aleve, Midol, Tylenol, and ibuprofen to push away the pain. Tam became deeply depressed and scrambled to take control of her body.

Disordered eating slowly crept into Tam's life. If she couldn't control the pain, then she could at least control what she consumed, she thought. Tam spent hours exercising, doing sit-ups, and practicing for varsity tennis. Her weight dropped and her periods stopped coming regularly. This made the stabbing pain in her abdomen subside, but she kept getting sicker. Eventually, Tam stopped playing sports because she'd pass out when the pain seared, from her womb to her gut. This was a period of extraordinary fear and confusion for Tam because she felt out of control: nobody could explain the pain, and few people believed her. A year later, she was hospitalized for anorexia and bulimia, weighing 69 pounds at five feet tall.[7]

When Tam was in the hospital, she met with a therapist who asked if she was molested. Tam refuted the molestation implication but described how emotional and verbal abuse from her parents and occasional physical abuse from her mother were persistent and often hidden (causing bruises on her back, neck, and stomach). She'd have constant ear infections, strep, and pneumonia too. Tam wonders if these infections were complicated by her mom's stress-induced chain smoking. As family business owners, her parents didn't have good health insurance or extra cash to foot the bill. The financial strain of Tam's infections and pain spun into a cycle of doubt that made Tam question herself: "You better be sick!" her parents would say. "It better be worth me taking time off work and bringing you to the doctor." Tam recalled, "Even now when I go to the doctor, I have a terrible fear they won't believe me. And I think that started when I was little."

When Tam left the hospital, she started to physically heal. She started taking birth control pills to control her pain. When she gained more weight, her periods came back. Her parents had moved while she was away, and a new school provided Tam space to reinvent herself. She also faced her first surgery for endometriosis, where they found more endometriosis deposits on her reproductive organs, colon, and bladder. They gave her Vicodin and Tylenol with codeine, and later OxyContin for the pain. She missed a lot of school.

When Tam recovered, she tried to make up for lost time. She joined a fast crowd in her new school, and things got tense fast with her parents. When the tension peaked, Tam's parents kicked her out, and she moved into a friend's trailer. Her parents eventually agreed to help her rent a room somewhere, and she started dating a friend from school. Soon after, he moved into the rented room with her, and after graduation, they married. But it didn't last long. Tam realized that what she thought was love was actually a possessive nature, and she resisted; he became abusive, and she left him. Through the divorce, she felt periods of safety that alternated with periods of insecurity.

BIOLOGY ENTANGLED

For centuries, endometriosis was referred to as a wandering uterus, suffocating womb, ovaritis, pelvic insanity, menstrual madness, and hysteria itself. It wasn't until the late 1880s that endometriosis was recognized and studied as a distinct disease, and until the 1920s that biological causes were identified as buried in the abdominal and obstetric pain and menstrual bleeding.[8] In 1927, a gynecologist at Albany Hospital named John Sampson used a microscope to examine biopsies of endometrial tissue growing cysts on and surrounding his patients' ovaries. Sampson coined the term *endometriosis* based on 293 cases he'd examined over a period of five years, theorizing that menstrual blood carried with it sloughed-off bits of tissue that flowed through the fallopian tubes and became implanted on the ovaries or perineum, causing extraordinary pain.[9] While this was a very clear explanation of what happens, the question remains: why? To this day, gynecologists call it "a riddle of etiology."[10]

Yet, endometriosis is extraordinarily common. It's estimated that one in ten women around the world experience endometriosis, and that it takes between six and ten years from one's first symptoms to be correctly diagnosed. Endometriosis is particularly hard to diagnose and therefore quite often unverifiable because it is characteristically hidden. It can start with the first menstrual period, which was most likely the case for Tam, and continue until or after menopause. This leads to inflammation and scar tissue forming in the pelvic region and (infrequently) beyond. This pain is unimaginable to someone who has never experienced it. Yet, over time, people like Tam build extraordinary pain thresholds, which make them delay care and live with disabling pain for years.

Endometriosis exemplifies what Nortin Hadler has called the "tyranny of torts" where people cannot get well if they are constantly trying to prove that they are sick.[11] A tort is a law meant to right a wrong. While issues of property disputes or personal injury are clear, the need to validate illness when there is no widely accepted set of biological markers, or *validation* of illness in the medical sense, makes showing proof nearly impossible. In the case of fibromyalgia, which is Hadler's focus, he argues that the contested illness is revealed in "widespread pain and peculiarly widespread tenderness when poked by the examiner," but rarely is there a biological marker that suits the clinician, and certainly not a judge determining disability.[12] Instead, "in absence of impairment, society is not prepared to believe them."[13] This is not unique to fibromyalgia but indeed a common feature of living with an unverifiable illness. However, as medical anthropologist Abigail Dumes reminds us, "medical unexplained illness is not a biomedical anomaly but, rather, a fundamental feature of biomedicine."[14]

Indeed, living with a shared experience of intense chronic pain is a fundamental characteristic of complex chronic conditions. In her book *Health Conditions*, philosopher Elizabeth Barnes muses on the fact that pain in essence is a distinguishing symptom of tissue damage, which can be a major cause of disability, be it episodic or consistent. People experience pain in different ways, for different reasons, and for varied durations. Barnes argues that chronic pain, which may persist after the tissue damage has healed, is experienced in such varied ways in part because of its "emotive aspect" that can be understood as "the sense in which the physical sensation is blended together with a sense of distress, distraction, or unpleasantness" and "is built into the very nature of pain."[15] Some of this pain can be explained by the indelible marks of oppression that have constructed such a difficult social environment for people living with a disability. While this framing incorporates the legacies of intergenerational violence as embedded in our bodies, memories, and subconscious, it also reveals the ways in which many people I've spoken to have felt unsafe, or described a lack of safety throughout their lives.[16] Because the emotional content of pain is, Barnes argues, so subjective, this aspect of suffering cannot be disentangled from the meaningful ways in which people experience the world. This may include pain linked to a traumatic or stressful experience of the past or fear for an unknown future, or frustration with the uncertainty of the present. These are not only individual experiences, but also disabilities that are, as feminist anthropologists Faye Ginsburg and Rayna Rapp have argued, deeply imbued in social relations, particularly in how families are configured, and possibly reconfigured when a beloved becomes ill.[17]

Grappling to control the bodymind is a common trope in psychological theory around eating disorders, and often antidepressants are used to manage these symptoms.[18] Jean-Martin Charcot and then his student Pierre Janet perceived anorexia and bulimia to be reflections of hysteria, arguing that when the psychogenic origins of these symptoms were cured (e.g., through hypnosis), then elements of hysteria (like anorexia) resolved. Both believed that such conditions were deeply rooted in past traumatic events and in regression to earlier developmental stages.[19] And, it's very likely Tam's health problems were deeply rooted in the life history that led her to this point. However, focusing exclusively on her socioemotional history overlooks the inherent physical nature of Tam's distress: the stabbing pain that recurred from her endometriosis and made her feel unsafe in her own bodymind. In *Gut Feminism*, Elizabeth Wilson argued, "The gut is sometimes angry, sometimes depressed, sometimes acutely self-destructive; under the stress of severe dieting, these inclinations come to dominate the gut's responsivity to the world. At these moments any radical distinction between stomach and mood, between vomiting and rage, is artificial."[20] Therapist and anthropologist Rebecca Lester has explained that some women diagnosed with anorexia "are convinced that physical fragility is the only reason other people pay attention to them or express concern for their well-being."[21] Hence, Tam may have felt the only way someone would take her pain seriously was if there was another more visible condition that legitimated her suffering.

This issue of safety is also crucial for understanding Tam's story. Hailey Lauer, a therapist and social worker who has worked in various inpatient and outpatient clinics, from prisoners to people suffering from addiction, told me, "Persistent pain and chronic stress are intimately connected, and pain is a safety mechanism. People who are in pain do not feel safe. They're afraid of their pain, and they're afraid of other things. And often when you dig into their life stories, they've never felt safe, or extreme things happened to them that destroyed their sense of safety. And then the pain follows." A Black American woman living with chronic illness explained to me how this is compounded by race: she said, "When I am not believed, I get flush and physically weak."

Stories like Tam's are often hidden within narratives of childhood violence that become intertwined with illness in adulthood. Some scholars have demonstrated how closely these adverse childhood events knit into chronic heart-linked diseases later in life.[22] When children endure such traumas in multiples, their thresholds for stabilization in the immune, endocrine, and nervous systems are irreversibly altered.[23] While such experiences can cause recurrent anxiety and depression, there are often deep-seated biological consequences that cascade from emotional trauma. These intimate biological connections also become social and political ones, where society ultimately frames how people are perceived and how they perceive living in a world that not only is sexist and patriarchal but also favors able-bodied people.

FINDING STRONGER GROUND

After a tumultuous childhood, Tam's life started to turn around. Tam enrolled in courses at a community college and finished at a small private college in St. Paul, working two jobs to get by. During this time, she studied in Morocco and separated her new life from her old life. Even as she started to flourish, she confronted traumas: she experienced sexual assault, and her sister died tragically in a car crash. To most people, this would appear extraordinary. Yet, Tam described to me how she was able to compartmentalize the pain, especially as she dove into a new relationship with Keith. Tam and Keith quickly became inseparable, and when Tam had to have another surgery, Keith convinced her to move in with him. Her pain had intensified so much from endometriosis, and Keith offered to nurse her through her recovery. During the surgery, they found more endometriosis deposits than they expected on her bladder, colon, and reproductive organs. They lasered them off, and she was hopeful she could finally recover with Keith's support.

In the years that followed, Tam's health stabilized, she finished college, and she married Keith. They moved to Tucson for her to study

Middle Eastern studies. They felt secure and settled for a short time—exceedingly happy together. However, things quickly began to unravel again. This time it was Keith: he was diagnosed with a brain tumor. They moved back to Minnesota for treatment. He lived for two more years.

During the entirety of Keith's sickness, Tam was well. She said, "When people are caregivers, they can't get sick. It's a protective mechanism." Keith died in August, and by December Tam's pain from her endometriosis surged again, unraveling the progress made in a stable time when her health was imperative to support Keith. Back in Tucson, Tam relied on their mutual friend Tylor, who brought a familiarity and stability to her life that made her feel more grounded and confident in a time of utter crisis. He also helped her administer a Lupron shot her gynecologist had prescribed to manage her tissue growth and lower risk for adhesions and scar tissue that might cause more pain during her next surgery. They caused constant hot flashes, night sweats, fatigue, and horrible mood swings. She also leaned on Tylor emotionally, and they began to fall in love.

Over the next several years, Tam finished her degree and moved to Beirut. Her life ebbed and flowed with intense sickness and incredible joy. She married Tylor and they built a happy life together. Tam had learned how to manage her pain, while dealing with kidney stones, endometriosis pain, and a fear that she might never have a baby. When she found out she was pregnant for the first time, she was shocked. Although she miscarried, she became hopeful of becoming a mother. Tam eventually had a healthy pregnancy and called Eli her miracle baby.

After the baby, Tam had a Mirena intrauterine device, a hormonal IUD, inserted to manage hormones, prevent pregnancy, and mitigate the pain. For nearly three years she had no periods, no pain, and felt strong. It was the healthiest she had been during her adult life, which she attributes to breastfeeding. It is not uncommon for people with endometriosis to have brief respites from endo pain during pregnancy and breastfeeding.[24] It is similarly not uncommon for people with autoimmune diseases, from lupus to Crohn's, to improve and possibly go into remission during these periods (however, it's variable and pregnancy can make some women sicker).[25] Tam became so passionate about breastfeeding that she became accredited as an International Board Certified Lactation Consultant (IBCLC) and founded the Mama 2 Mama Beirut Breastfeeding support group. When Eli was weaned, however, her pain came back.

This was ten years ago. Tam was rushed to the emergency room with a combination of abdominal pain, chills, and fever. They told her it was gastroenteritis and sent her home. For a few months, the fever came and went, but the pain in her gut stayed; she started her old strategies of alternating acetaminophen and ibuprofen for the pain. Back in Tucson, Tam scoured her medical records and saw one doctor had questioned whether her pain could be linked to a uterine perforation. The doctor removed the IUD, but Tam's pain remained: she couldn't eat or drink, had bloody stools, and was completely bedridden. One day, her pain was so intense, her father-in-law rushed her to the ER, where she was given pain meds and a referral for a colonoscopy.

Looking back, Tam's enteric nervous system dysregulation, clinically diagnosed as ulcerative colitis—a form of irritable bowel syndrome, or IBS—could reflect the depth of stress and trauma she has carried over her life course combined with the hormonal changes associated with removing the IUD. Some patients call this the "Mirena crash," which has been measurably difficult for some people, and Tam described it as unusually difficult because of her history of inflammatory disease.

A year later, they were back in Beirut, and Tam visited her gastrointestinal doctor. She was relieved to see him because Tam found sharing her complicated story with new clinicians was often demoralizing. She regularly faced skepticism about whether her story and symptoms were real. Her trusted doctor in Beirut said her pain wasn't from ulcerative colitis but rather an acute colitis infection that was so bad it looked chronic (and resembled an autoimmune disease). After several other tests, they removed some polyps and started her on gabapentin (a nerve pain medication meant to calm down her neuropathy—it's a common drug for shingles, epilepsy, and multiple sclerosis). Eli was three, and that whole year she was bedridden.

Tam considers her laparoscopy for endometriosis the following year to be her last, even though it was two consecutive embolization procedures, where they cauterize the vascular networks to the endometrial tissue. The pain was "indescribable," but the surgeries alleviated the pain, and she began to recover. It was also when her doctors diagnosed her with pelvic congestion syndrome, which provided some legitimacy for her constant aches and pains in that area.

The next year Tam had a complete hysterectomy and thought medical trauma was finally behind her. Then, her mast cells started acting up. Mast cells are a type of white blood cell found throughout the body that helps control immune responses, including those to certain bacteria and parasites.[26] The mast cells release chemicals like histamines, heparin, cytokines, and growth factors. The chemicals are released during allergic reactions or certain immune responses. One example of this is the cytokine storms that have been widely referenced biological responses to COVID-19, resulting in several key pro-inflammatory cytokines that can relate to disease severity.[27]

Tam was diagnosed with mast cell activation syndrome, which can cause flushing, itching, abdominal pain, diarrhea, hypotension, syncope, and musculoskeletal pain.[28] These features are the result of mast cell mediator release and infiltration into target organs. The doctor prescribed steroids, which might have caused her adrenal glands to stop making cortisol on their own. Although steroids helped with one symptom, they caused her to gain seventy pounds and develop severe immune dysregulation. In other words, her body shut down. This type of cause and effect is not unusual for people living with a complex chronic illness.

It's nearly impossible to determine where Tam's diagnostic odyssey began and ended. Certainly, her central diagnosis is her endometriosis, but along the way she's managed so many social and traumatic stressors as well as several biological sirens of distress. Today Tam takes twenty-five pills a day, including a cocktail of mast cell stabilizers and an assortment of other medication. She organizes this labyrinth of medication in a large multicolored pill case that is both tasteful and joyful. Based on her own patient networks and years of experience, she is also investigating new therapies.

A few years ago, Tam, Tylor, and Eli moved to Ireland. Now, in a coastal town outside of Dublin, Tam has cultivated a new normal. The temperate weather and reliable healthcare system have improved Tam's health immensely. She continues to manage health disruptions through medication, regulation of emotions, social relations, and environment. She's built a dynamic community of friends and feels she has some control over her health—even though living well each day is a constant journey. Tam's new normal involves being thoughtful about every place she goes, efforts she can expend each day, and people she interacts with, from everyday chats at her son's school to advocacy with clinicians and policymakers. She continues to engage with international breastfeeding groups and has become a lay expert in rare diseases.

DISABLED ECOLOGIES

Sunaura Taylor argues in *Disabled Ecologies: Lessons from a Wounded Desert* that recognizing how to manage and live with injury and sickness requires that we situate people's lived experience within society and think through the political systems that make it so very hard to live with disability. Using the phrase "environmentalism of the injured" recognizes how the struggles people navigate with disability are deeply rooted in the systems of care—from social relations to health systems and financial support. Just as microbiomes can shift through manipulation, Taylor suggests, ecological and social systems can transform in a way that resembles how organisms can "mutate, evolve, be harmed, and also heal."[29]

Thinking in terms of multiplicity or thresholds is not common in medicine or health systems more generally. Often in medicine, thinking in terms of comorbidity or even multimorbidity is perceived as pushing the envelope. However, it's impossible to think about the lived experience of complex chronic illness without thinking in terms of entanglements of multiple things. Feminist theorist Elizabeth Wilson suggests in her book *Gut Feminism* that a more dynamic schema for digestion, respiration, antiperistalsis, neurotransmitters, and mood is essential to understand how multiple conditions build on one another. Even when these connections are not immediately visible in the clinical data, she contends, that these links between mind and body, psyche and soma, are much more deeply entangled than many believe. Wilson is not arguing that organs are indistinguishable (that would preclude her from teaching in any medical school). Rather, she claims that "there is no originary demarcation between these entities; they are always already coevolved and coentangled."[30] Such thinking is an even more important point when we think about the gut as the "second brain" because of the network of nerves that regulate the gut. The enteric nervous system therefore cannot be dissociated from thoughts, feelings, or disturbance in other parts of the nervous system that may trigger dysregulation.[31]

Thus, there needs to be an understanding that chronic pains, particularly in the gut, are not only cultural or biological problems but also ecological ones. The gut is directly linked to the mouth, which is a central way in which the outside world travels into our bodies. These travelers then encounter small ecosystems through and around the body—from the mouth to the gut and the skin. These infections pile up and interact within the environments in which they reside, which are often called microbiomes. Microbiomes are the combinations of viruses, bacteria, fungi, and their genes that sit within in the body. The gut microbiome is a good metaphor for interaction with the external world, in part because it is an opening to it, engulfing and internalizing the external world around us.[32] While microbiomes are often deemed a biological framework, thinking about how the invaders become part of our bodyminds also pushes us to think somewhat differently about disability and how dis-abled people navigate a disabling world. Ill-health is always embedded in our social environments as well as "intermeshed" when our environments become inseparable from the bodies we inhabit.[33]

Thresholds, then, may spill over when certain microbiomes come in contact with invaders like viruses, bacteria, parasites, or trauma, revealing themselves somewhat in the gut but obfuscated by the social and political chaos of a pandemic.[34] This is even more provocative if we accept that the gut, brain, skin, and other tissues have differentiated microbiomes throughout the body. Many of the people living with a complex chronic health condition whom I spoke to for this project carefully described to me how they managed the excruciating pain that surged in their guts, at different moments throughout their illness, with careful diets to reduce inflammation and control the pain, just as Tam attempted to manage her pain by withholding food. Bethany, for example, whose story opened the book, described how she intervened in a squeaky gut by consuming a restricted set of foods, like celery, peanut butter, and herbal tea, and fasting roughly every other day, seeking to calm the agitation. It worked, but it took several months for her to rekindle equilibrium.

The threshold metaphor can also be useful when thinking about how chronic stress may impact the body and the brain differently within and between people. Neuroscientist Bruce McEwen, who studies how stress hormones reshape neural circuits and brain structures, has theorized that allostatic loads may appear different from person to person, linking to both social and pathogenic causes.[35] On the one hand, this may be a result of microbiomes that ultimately mediate how stress interacts with the brain and body. However, existing vulnerabilities, such as co-infections (particularly from the herpes family viruses), immune dysregulation, and a persistence of inflammation, often play a fundamental role in pushing thresholds into indeterminable dysregulation when a bodymind confronts an unrelenting invader, such as SARS-CoV-2.[36]

Theories abound about what fuels long COVID, and where the specific triggers may lie. Many of these theories focus on a certain trigger point that may dysregulate the body on a large scale, and then this dysregulation is amplified in multiple systems at once. Mike VanElzakker, a neuroscientist at Harvard, proposed a theory to explain post-viral conditions that serves as a good example of this. In 2013, VanElzakker argued in *Medical Hypotheses* that the vagus nerve is possibly the key to ME/CFS symptoms, in part because it tricks the body into thinking it's sick. The term *vagus* shares the same root as *vagabond*, which means "wandering" in Latin, which makes good sense because the vagus nerve serves as the highway into and out of the brain.[37] The vagus nerve's highly branched nerve bundles control involuntary bodily functions like digestion, heart rate, and immune function, making the vagus the largest nerve in the body. However, it is also closely tied to the outside world and likely to encounter pathogens.[38]

Originally focused on understanding the neurobiology of trauma, VanElzakker was drawn to study ME/CFS when a close friend became so sick, she had to leave law school. He dove into untangling possible biological pathways to explain her suffering. In the case of ME/CFS, VanElzakker argues, the virus tricks the vagal nerve into thinking the body is sick, which triggers immune cells to release proinflammatory cytokines that send a signal to the brain that the body is sick.[39] This is not unlike the well-documented cytokine response storm associated with the acute virus of COVID-19.[40] Many larger studies suggest a similar pathophysiology of vagus nerve dysfunction in people living with long COVID.[41] In these cases, vagal nerve disruptions are linked to defining symptoms of dysautonomia: digestion problems, heart rate and blood pressure, immune function, mood, muscle aches, itching, and problems with speech, smell, and tastes.[42] This theory is also referred to, in circles of neuroscientists trying to disentangle theories around long COVID, as *a theory of crucial nerve damage*.[43] However, VanElzakker described to me how pivotal microbiomes may be for understanding why people with long COVID get so sick and so differently. [44] Indeed, it may be not only nerve damage but also the multiplicity of viruses and bacteria that cultivate small ecosystems that may affect certain systems differently within and between people.

Others suggest that similar triggers are amplified by epigenetics—a theory that external forces (like viruses) might activate certain genes without changing people's DNA.[45] Maureen Hanson, a developmental biologist at Cornell University who spent most of her career untangling the mystery of ME/CFS, recently argued that immune cells called T cells, which work against pathogens, dysregulate and cause cells and bodies to feel perpetually fatigued.[46] These are the same biological disruptors that cause fatigue in cancer patients, and there are existing treatments for them. Hanson and her team argue that epigenetics may be a central part of *why* some people experience disabling fatigue and others do not. Yet, these pathologies do not map onto every person diagnosed with post-viral conditions the same way: some people's illness may follow different pathways, such as via the vascular or respiratory systems.[47]

As Elizabeth Wilson argues in her book *Psychosomatic*, the biological underpinnings of these symptoms have been dismissed for too long, even though we know that an interaction of multiple factors makes the bodymind so absolutely inflamed. The truth is, there is no concrete explanation that has been widely accepted to explain complex chronic conditions, including long COVID. And, by thinking in terms of thresholds, we can understand why there might not be one pathway that can or should explain every case. The concept of thresholds enables us to sit within the gray areas of health and disease. In many cases, the medical history is so complicated that the revisionists have a difficult time interpreting what was biological or psychological, felt or perceived, real or unreal. However, the fact of the matter is that everything, be it a virus, parasite, trauma, bacterium, chemical, or a unique interaction among these invaders, is affecting people in deep ways that may not be measurable but are at work deep within the bodymind.

PART TWO

POLITICS

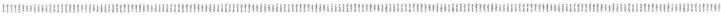

5

DISABLING CULTURE

||||||||||||||||||||||||||||||||||||||||||||||||||||||||||||||||||||||||||||||||||||||||||||||||||||||||||||||||||||||||||||||||||||||||||||||||||||||||||||||||||||||||||||||||||||||

I GOT COVID IN EARLY January of 2023. I believe I caught it on an international flight when I was masked. I had never tested positive for COVID-19 before and wondered whether I might have already had it. It would be impossible not to have ever had it, I thought, after constant exposures at work. I was pinged weekly that I had a positive COVID exposure in one of my classrooms at Georgetown University. I must have been asymptomatic, I convinced myself.

My acute illness experience was pretty standard. I spent nights on end coughing, but I never feared that I couldn't breathe. I felt complete exhaustion and lay in bed for days. My symptoms were summed up by intense malaise, fever, coughing, and brain fog.

I tested positive for two weeks, but the coughing stopped and fever broke in a week. The brain fog and chronic fatigue lingered for months. I kept texting my friends to see how long they felt this tired. Most said a couple weeks, others said a few months. Oh no, I thought, this might settle in for a long time.

A couple weeks after I was back at work, a new symptom crept up: my old friend anxiety became as intense as my fatigue. I attributed the anxiety to everything I was juggling: teaching an overload, volunteering, unfinished writing, and taxiing my elementary school children around. My mood continued to deteriorate, and I realized that I was having more days when I felt anxious and sad than when I didn't. These roller-coaster moods reminded me of the postpartum depression I had after giving birth to my youngest daughter.

By the end of February, I met with my family nurse practitioner. Although my general anxiety ebbs and flows in accordance with the (im)balance of parenting-work-family-life, I realized post-COVID anxiety was something different. Mine was deeply entwined with depression and a constant feeling of lack of control. Things started to balance out once I started taking antianxiety medication and shifted my time around to make space for more self-care.

It was not long after I started interviewing people with long COVID that I realized how common an escalation of anxiety and depression is for people who've had COVID. I read research studies that suggested that those who had more intense anxious and depressive responses after getting COVID-19 were also people who were more vulnerable to anxiety and depression before infection.[1] Bethany (whose story opened the book) had told me, "Our sympathetic nervous system is stuck in the fight-or-flight mode, since I stay so jumpy and nervous all the time." This can be explained by the simplest stress response: when a stressor is over, and the stress response turns off, your parasympathetic nervous system is supposed to calm down your body.[2] This system of checks and balances is disrupted when the virus pushes us over a threshold.

After four months, I started to feel better. I still crash with intense fatigue after some prolonged exertions, such as a long trip or intense combined work-caregiving schedule, which was rarely the case before infection. However, my long COVID story is a mild one compared with so many others. For instance, a year before my infection, a bright student of mine came down with a much more severe form of long COVID.

A CULTURE OF PRODUCTIVITY

Nearly two years after the COVID-19 pandemic began, Ken Kaplan went to a party. It had been months since he'd seen childhood friends—mostly outside and distanced—and years since he'd been to a party. When we went into quarantine, a family member got very sick, which required him to be especially careful whenever he left the house: masking and avoiding stores at busy times. However, eighteen months into the pandemic, life seemed to get back to normal, and he was invited to a small New Year's Eve gathering. He thought to himself, It will be a small group of vaccinated friends, and they understand how careful I've been. When he arrived unmasked, people kept swarming into the house party. He thought, Who are these people, and are they even vaccinated? He let his vigilance slip. He got sick two days later.

Ken got really sick. He quarantined from his family in his garage and set up telehealth visits with his general practitioner, Dr. P. By the end of January, Dr. P diagnosed him with long COVID based on his symptoms: constant brain fog, intermittent headaches, devastating chronic fatigue, body aches everywhere, on-and-off-again nausea and vomiting, unexpected dizziness and syncope (where he would randomly pass out), loss of taste and smell, shortness of breath, and memory loss. Ken was relieved when the university delayed inviting students back in person until the end of January. He was able to join the first couple weeks of lectures virtually as he navigated his fevers and forced himself to complete the readings through his brain fog and malaise. What became apparent to Ken was that he had a difficult time not only reading the words, but also retaining the content. How am I going to get through the semester? he thought. Never did he seriously consider taking a leave of absence—he pushed on.

A year later, Ken sat on a red couch in my office and explained the varied ways in which his brain fog manifested, ebbing and flowing over the first eighteen months of illness. Shortly before returning to school in February, I had discussed with Ken that he might take a leave of absence. Ken thought he could continue by focusing on the bare minimum. I recommended that Ken start journaling about his long COVID journey—writing every day about his feelings, physical symptoms, experiences, and observations. This culminated in an honors thesis about his personal journey living with long COVID while interviewing other patients, clinicians, academics, and policymakers to understand why—at the time—people weren't taking it seriously. Despite this incredible achievement, I would argue, one reason Ken wouldn't take a break from school to recover from his illness was because doing so would run up against the culture of achievement he was navigating in the university.

Living in a cultural context characterized by productivity and efficiency is what makes surviving a condition characterized by disabling fatigue and memory inconsistency particularly challenging.[3] Novelist Florence King has called our cultural obsession the "American way of stress." She wrote that "stress has become a status symbol," making people feel "busy, important, and in demand, and simultaneously deprived, ignored, and victimized. Stress makes them feel interesting and complex instead of boring and simple."[4] While this critique extends well beyond illness, it demonstrates how a normalization of pushing through, despite illness, might be perceived as a cultural badge of honor in American society. It may be that such a notion, while frequent in academia and medicine, cultivates distrust of patients who express disabling fatigue.

Anthropologist Neely Myers has made a similar argument in her book *Breaking Points* that emphasizes how such expectations are particularly difficult for young people. Myers argues that what makes this time difficult is that young people are navigating moral agency, or the ability to be seen as a good person by those around them. When a culture is defined by productivity and efficiency, these norms frame how people conceive of their autobiographic power as well as notions of being "good enough" for and in relation to the people in their orbit.[5]

This cultural conscience is deeply rooted in capitalism and its bedfellow, misogyny. American journalist Ed Yong wrote in *The New York Times*, "As energy-depleting illnesses that disproportionately affect women, long COVID and M.E./C.F.S. are easily belittled by a sexist society that trivializes women's pain, and a capitalist one that values people according to their productivity."[6] This framing also harkens back to George Beard's framing of neurasthenia and the problem with Americanitis. In this way, long COVID has revisited a conversation of what it means to be part of the cultural fabric of America when one's engine becomes depleted, and one's sense of American-ness begins to unravel.

BRAIN FOG MULTIPLE

"This isn't a fog," Ken wrote in his journal during his fourth month of living with long COVID. "This is life under an ice sheet. The term *brain fog* has everyone I meet expecting I'll be better any day now. Like a morning cloud layer temporarily obscuring a photo op of the Golden Gate Bridge. I need people to understand that this is debilitating and varied. It isn't just going to disappear, and its progression isn't linear."

For Ken, it was possibly his memory inconsistencies, often characterized as brain fog, that were the most difficult symptoms for him to navigate while he was in school. Brain fog has been understood as several things: confusion, trouble concentrating, anxiety, forgetting, and even headaches.[7] The term *brain fog* has been applied to nearly anything associated with the mind when someone experiences an unverifiable illness, and it is an exceedingly common symptom. When someone feels hazy, tired, and distracted, it's called brain fog. Yet, when fatigue remains and memory goes intermittently, many people call that brain fog.[8]

Ken's memory was inconsistent, but it was the social dynamics that were the most difficult part. Struggling to remember things in ten-minute intervals made it incredibly difficult to focus on things that usually made up a central part of his identity, such as being a good student. However, he would avoid social interactions with friends because he felt too sick to show up or worried that his friends would be disappointed when he couldn't follow the conversations or engage like he once did. He found these social interactions exhausting and needed to save energy for his schoolwork. Ken's personality became slower and quieter. He felt self-conscious about explaining to others what was going on with him, shying away and saying everything was fine.

Anthropologist Emily Lim Rogers has argued that for many people brain fog becomes "real" when it becomes social—and when their "fogginess" is not dismissed but rather legitimized.[9] It took several weeks for Ken to have his academic accommodations approved. Even still, two professors made it clear that they didn't believe him (while two others were incredibly understanding). Living through this experience made Ken take other people's fogginess much more seriously because he realized how invisible and alone this experience can make you feel, especially when you are surrounded by people.

LEGITIMIZING FOGGINESS

Part of the confusion is that the concept of brain fog captures too much. The fog itself differs significantly for many people. In the most serious cases, people's symptoms are life-changing and disabling so that they cannot function in a way that they might have before and as a result must adapt to new ways of living. For others, brain fog is mostly word recall and forgetfulness.

Most people I've spoken to living with serious symptoms don't call it brain fog. Instead, many emphasize that they have experienced brain injury. This framework is not unfounded. Studies suggest that some people have long-term brain injuries a year after contracting SARS-CoV-2, validated by cognitive tests, symptoms, brain scans, and biomarkers.[10] These studies hypothesize that brain injury from infections might age someone twenty years. However, these symptoms are not all that different from those from a bump, blow, or jolt to the head or hit to the body that rapidly moves the brain back and forth so that it bounces or twists. With an observed blow to the head, we might identify this as a concussion or traumatic brain injury. My friend Amir Babaei-Mahani, an internist, described this to me as a "brain shake." Think of your brain as sitting in a hard box, he said. If you shake it in that hard box, then the brain might warp out of shape. It's fine in every way after the injury, but there may be weird cognitive issues that linger. While the immediate and lingering impacts of an acute hit are obvious, rarely do people conceive of infections in the same way.

Yet, for nearly four centuries, syphilis was a common infection perceived to be the main cause of dementia.[11] *Dementia* is a general term to describe people's inability to remember, think, or make decisions; biologically, dementia looks like a loss of neurons and axonal connections linked to neurodegeneration. This inevitably interferes with doing things that, before illness, people would have called routine. With effective medication, however, syphilis is rarely linked to dementia today. Instead, it's generally accepted that one in ten people will experience some form of dementia after retirement age and that one in three elders will have dementia when they reach the age of eighty.[12]

Infections caused by Epstein-Barr, herpes, influenza, pneumonia, syphilis, HIV, Lyme, Zika, Ebola, SARS, dengue, and West Nile also demonstrate powerful links to cognitive declines, particularly when people experience multiple infections at once. A study of thousands of people in Finland found that a person with viral encephalitis (brain inflammation) was thirty times more likely to develop memory loss than someone without.[13] Yet, many of these infections may not be progressive in nature, meaning that an overactive immune response or degradation and dysregulation of nerve cells may cause short-term or episodic declines in memory.[14] Memory is rarely an isolated symptom with COVID. People also experience fatigue, fog, and sleep trouble. One in four have memory troubles like Ken. Some get raging headaches.[15] In many ways, chronic living for people in the wake of viral infection can ebb and flow in extremely unpredictable ways.

So many people felt their loved ones couldn't understand what they were going through. A grandmother who had lived with epilepsy most of her life described it this way: "I feel like I'm living entire days and weeks of my life in that postictal epileptic haze. I'm drowsy and confused, usually with splitting migraines. But I've had to start telling people I'm having epileptic episodes when I'm struggling with brain fog because they believe epilepsy is real. Telling the truth and saying I'm dealing with brain fog is more work than it's worth."

In retrospect, Ken thinks he should have taken a leave of absence from school when his symptoms were the worst. Yet, he never considered it. Ken's desire to become a physician drove his perseverance—he worried missing a semester of science courses would get him off-track for medical school. This type of self-imposed pressure is fueled by a normative pressure to perform at an unsustainable level that was compromised further by Ken's tendency to push hard and then crash. It exemplifies how the social and material conditions of the university "'dis-able' the full participation of a variety of minds and bodies."[16]

JO'S STORY

Vox Jo Hsu's been chronically ill since they were twenty. I reached out to Jo because I read some interesting opinion pieces they had written on racism and long COVID as a trans Asian American disabled scholar.

When they first became sick, it was a somewhat typical case. There was an acute virus that lasted for weeks and wouldn't go away. Then they got better. Then they got sick again. "It was like I was trapped into this continual cycle," Jo said. They thought, How am I possibly catching the same bug over and over again?

Jo went to graduate school for creative writing and felt somewhat normal. It wasn't until Jo was in their late twenties, and when they'd begun their first tenure-track academic job, when things started to unravel. For years Jo was a CrossFit enthusiast. Suddenly every workout made them spiral: workouts would leave them drained and require rest for hours and sometimes days. The doctor told Jo that these symptoms triggered by exercise were not a medical problem.

Jo explained that two years later "it got really bad where if I exercised, or if my heart rate went up above resting threshold, I would be sort of immobile for a long period. And that was when I was resistant to the idea that I had ME because all I knew about were the stereotypes. I knew enough to know that this was not only heavily stigmatized, but also under-researched and under-resourced. So, if I had ME, there would be no treatment for it. So, I thought, please literally anything but this."

This was an incredibly frustrating time in Jo's life. They posted a rant about their symptoms on Facebook, and a close friend gently reached out: "Have you considered that you might have ME?" Jo's friend had been diagnosed with ME/CFS years ago, and she approached it like an academic, sending Jo a full Google Doc with a bibliography of resources. Jo just started going through it and thought, Shit, this is probably it.

Today Jo Hsu is a professor at the University of Texas at Austin, where they study the political and embodied impact of storytelling, focusing on how narratives shape policy, social norms, and personal and public health. Jo writes about how discriminatory stories infiltrate medical research, and how this research gets interpreted and causes harm. This wasn't what Jo was originally working on, however. Jo remembers a transformational moment when they served on a panel for a screening of the documentary film *Unrest* by Jennifer Brea.[17] When Brea was told again and again that her sickness was *all in her head*, she turned her camera on herself to demonstrate the debilitating experience of the illness. Brea illustrates the agony of her debilitating fatigue, showing firsthand what it looks like to quite literally not be able to lift her physical body from the bed or walk up a flight of stairs.

What was meaningful to Jo was that it was the first time they'd seen a representation of anything that "wasn't the sort of caricature that is like white upper-middle-class 'yuppie flu,' the general stereotype. This was when these things came together and started to really sink in." Like the stereotype, Brea was a Harvard University graduate student working toward her PhD when this illness took over her physical body. However, Brea spoke from the perspective of a Black and multiracial woman—and from the perspective of a researcher, driven to find her own evidence when the "experts" met the limits of their own knowledge. The very different light that Brea cast on the illness narrative had an impact on Jo. When her symptoms improved, Brea also interviewed others in video calls and eventually in person for the documentary *Unrest*. Through this work, Brea also founded the advocacy organization called #MEAction.

Jo looked into the condition, and it started to make sense. At the time Jo discovered the film *Unrest*, they were already working a tenure-track academic position. Jo said, "I wanted hard answers, and I finally had a job where I could afford it. I went to the Institute for Neuro-Immune Medicine in Florida." Jo spent around $1,500 between the appointment cost, travel, and hotel. The doctor told Jo, You have what you think you do, so you should rest. Jo was frustrated by this response, in part because rest is "so much easier as a concept than it is in practice."

Jo explained, "I'm one of the people who gets to be fully employed. So my energy envelope is much bigger than most people's, and I'm very fortunate in that way." Unlike some people with ME/CFS, Jo can continue with meaningful work that ensures some financial stability, although they carefully monitor their energy in ways that make sense day-to-day. In academia, Jo has the freedom to rearrange their schedule in a way that makes it a bit more adaptable, making it easier to manage chronic symptoms of fatigue, distraction, and muscle aches. Many people I've spoken to relied on government disability allowances, such as Supplemental Security Income—monthly payments for the elderly and people living with disabilities who have little to no resources. Many ended up relying on these services for years, in part because they couldn't continue working in environments that did not accommodate their disabilities.

ME/CFS differs in symptoms and severities over time and between people. This isn't uncommon for complex chronic conditions, or disabilities more generally, which are experienced and embodied differently among people and within families.[18] For instance, many people struggle to sleep, staying awake all night due to anxiety, restless legs, or numbness. Others struggle with memory, from short-term to long-term, and there is a variance in what types of memory and confusion people experience. While some people may present with a form of dementia, others struggle with word recall. Many people feel pain in the joints and the muscles and experience migraines or constant headaches. Some people experience night sweats. While some people experience depression, and many clinicians find this a defining feature of ME/CFS, many patients argue that their illness is more somatic and social in nature. This framing works against a common and harmful phrase mentioned by clinicians (either directly or indirectly) that ME/CFS is "all in your head."[19]

Jo contends that such "arguments enter a cultural context where disabled people are already treated with suspicion, and where psychiatric diagnoses are already weaponized to invalidate a person's self-knowledge. Let me be clear," Jo emphasized as I watched from the back of an auditorium where they delivered a speech to scientists at a National Institutes of Health meeting in early December of 2023, "whether or not you actually believe a discriminatory narrative, your words can endorse it—with all the authority of your position."[20]

Yet, for people like Jo, who have a milder form of ME/CFS, which for them looks like chronic episodes of mononucleosis, acutely stressful or traumatic incidents can lay them up for days. For others, with a severe form of ME/CFS, exertions like taking a shower or walking for one minute on a treadmill can cause extraordinary post-exertional malaise exacerbation.

In the *Huffington Post*, Jo described how an incident of racist violence—in this case an aggressive verbal attack in a parking lot by a white woman—was the last straw that tipped them into a crash during what might have been an ordinary day. They explained, "The experience differs from patient to patient, but for me, physical and emotional stress provoke muscle weakness, lightheadedness, cognitive difficulty and days of full-body aches, crushing fatigue and digestive dysfunction. My sight and hearing also become hypersensitive, so that each glimmer of light is a bonfire. This woman's voice was a bludgeon."[21] While it took several days for Jo to recover physically, the weight of a history of homophobia, transphobia, anti-Asian racism, and violence persevered through this woman's hateful words. This was during the COVID-19 pandemic, amid surges of anti-Asian violence. Jo wrote, "Public suffering has always found scapegoats in marginalized communities."[22]

Before the pandemic shuttered businesses and kept people out of the classroom, Jo had begun to stabilize. It was the acute SARS-CoV-2 infection that reevoked Jo's unraveling, bringing them back to a state of illness that they had not experienced for some time. For Jo, the first infection "exacerbated the ME that I already had, but the post-exertional malaise is my worst symptom. It's the most frustrating one, but also the brain fog, lightheadedness, and digestive disruptions." Jo explained how long COVID manifests in a deepening of their existing illness, worsening fatigue, introducing full body aches, muscle pain, and most frustratingly, a regression of illness they had for some time managed with relative stability.

Despite Jo's scientific research, patient activism, and years living with their condition, they still don't feel like their knowledge is legitimated within clinical spaces. This is largely because they are consistently dismissed in clinical spaces, by medical societies, and within media reflections of people whose lives have been undone by illness. Jo told me, "If you cannot imagine me as a person you should care about, then there is no instinctive pathway to a relationship that can help me recover." Pushing the boundaries of how people—from the clinic to the streets—recognize who gets sick with complex chronic conditions and how to care for them is a constant social project that is deeply embedded in the disability movement.

A DIFFERENT KIND OF FATIGUE

Some of the most powerful moments in the film *Unrest* are Jennifer Brea's intimate portrayals of her physical manifestation of fatigue that is quite different from typical malaise. Most people I spoke to describe the difficulty of doing what before their illness were simple tasks, like taking a shower, walking to the mailbox, or picking up groceries. Many people also mentioned that not every day is the same. The intensity of exhaustion fluctuates through time, and many people prevent flare-ups by pacing—meaning treading carefully with their energy and moving through life in a way to engage meaningfully while protecting their well-being. The disability community calls this "crip time," which Ginsburg and Rapp argue defies "the assumed unproblematic linearity and pace of normate life, ignoring the time, energy, or resources required by people with disabilities."[23]

While I argue here that the experience of pushing through fatigue and finding a new way to navigate life in a culture of overwork and productivity is culturally constructed, it's important to recognize that the experience of fatigue is a global phenomenon. Nearly one in four people worldwide experience some fatigue, and one in ten experience some form of disabling fatigue that lasts more than six months and therefore is considered chronic.[24] While chronic fatigue syndrome afflicts more adults than children, it does affect the young, including more than one in 100 adolescents.[25]

Fatigue is not something attributed to one thing. In clinical contexts, fatigue is understood based on duration, severity, and a constellation of other diagnoses.[26] In life, fatigue is imbued in complex social relationships, emotional pain, somatic symptoms, and biological memories. In this way, not only fatigue, but also post-exertional malaise permeates chronic living through the rhythms of a new life of exertion and recovery. This is one aspect that Brea so beautifully demonstrates in *Unrest*, where her husband and others support her movement and rest through time—a dynamic that is constantly in flux. Pacing therefore becomes an essential element of chronic living, where people strategically manage their energy envelopes throughout the day.

Many people use spoon theory to manage their daily pacing. This metaphor—created by Christine Miserandino, who has lupus—conveys the idea that you begin the day with twelve spoons, which represents your energy for that day.[27] For most people, waking up and getting ready for the day takes one spoon, going to work takes four spoons, and they don't use all their spoons and they have some left at the end of the day. But people with energy-limiting illnesses need to think about their energy differently. For instance, getting out the door is four spoons, and going to work is six spoons. Then, doing an activity for a PTA meeting is four spoons, and going home to make dinner is another four spoons. This doesn't add up—and they just don't have the energy. Therefore, people living with ME/CFS think carefully about what they need to do throughout the day with pacing. Spoon theory is a helpful social tool too, conveying to loved ones that you need to rest:

"I'm sorry that I cannot do [the activity]; I only have two spoons left." One person joked, "Some days I don't have enough spoons and don't give a fork!"

Others use creative tactics to manage their symptoms. Jennifer Fricas, a professor living in Seattle, discovered several tricks to manage her symptoms and continue to live her life at a different pace. Fricas described post-exertional malaise as a "disproportionate crash of energy, fatigue, exhaustion, and many people get muscle weakness that is almost to the point of paralysis and that lasts for hours to weeks, depending on the level of exertion." When this started inhibiting her life, she turned to the digital #MEAction network to share information about symptoms and strategies to manage them. Based on the advice she gathered from others living with similar symptoms, she started using a power wheelchair to travel long distances, such as from the parking lot at work to her office across campus. Fricas calls her wheelchair a fundamental "prevention tool." This is because she is an ambulatory wheelchair user, meaning she can walk. Fricas uses the wheelchair to prevent exhaustion, conserve energy, and keep that energy for other activities, which increases her energy envelope throughout the day. Fricas knows that she won't live with the same energy levels she might have had before she got sick; however, she's reimagined a future living her life in a new light, at a different pace.

I spoke to Canadian physician Jennifer Hulme, who has written about how she found a peace with her new way of living, after chasing several theories. She wrote, "I am trying to come to a place of acceptance. I still hope to escape chronic symptoms, but I have found other people's stories validating and helpful; I want to help do that for others. I have seen one of the world experts on this subject, and the only thing we know helps is rest and pacing. I am taking more time off work. This is very, very hard for me to do as it is so much of my identity and source of joy and purpose. I am buying earphones to help with my neurological symptoms." She continued, "But save your money, except the antihistamine" (which can aid in some recovery), because care can be costly. Instead, she explained, "I am trying to be patient, as so many others are, waiting for solutions in the shadows as this 'acute on chronic' phase of the pandemic rages on."[28] In other words, the way the medical model doggedly and narrowly envisions cure can threaten to obscure the wisdom of people's bodies. Instead, they need to listen to their intuition and somatic needs because they know what it's really like to live with a dynamic disability and what may truly make a difference for their lives as they are.

6

THE RISE OF PATIENT
ACTIVISM

||||||||||||||||||||||||||||||||||||||||||||||||||||||||||||||||||||||||||||||||||||||||||||||||||||||||||||||||||||||||||||||||||||||||||||||||||||||

MANY PEOPLE WHO ARE ABLE-BODIED cannot imagine how difficult it is to live in a world that is so obsessed with efficiency
and productivity when one is not able-bodied. Susan Wendell described this challenge as the "able-bodied paradigm of
humanity," which relies on an idealized view of the human
bodymind as young, healthy, fit, and energized.[1] It is through
this idealization that the construct of disability is formed. In
this way, disability is not a biological problem. Instead,
disability becomes a struggle that people face within an
environment that does not provide accessibility to moving
and living in that world. Ginsburg and Rapp describe in their
work on "disability worlds" how disability is something that
is socially constructed within a certain environment. They
explain, "This paradigm insists that disability is not simply
lodged in the body but created by the social and material
conditions that 'dis-able' the full participation of a variety of
minds and bodies. Disability is thus recognized as the result

of negative interactions between a person with an impairment and his or her social environment."[2] This is why disability may be defined differently between contexts based on the people, places, landscapes, and technologies.

Disability scholar Amy Kenny told me, "The disabling environment makes it difficult for people to thrive." Kenny described how at places like Georgetown University, where we both work, a disabling culture of productivity is compounded by social and academic pressures that make everyday life difficult for someone living with a chronic illness. This is not unlike how a culture that resists incorporating ramps, elevators, automatic doors, and signage to access these points causes people relying on wheelchairs to feel less safe and accepted. She also reminded me that people living with anxiety (like me) might find anxiety medications to be an "access point." This is particularly salient when people are juggling intense pressures at work with caregiving for children, parents, and others. Similarly, someone who experiences post-exertional malaise might use a wheelchair as an access point to better manage their environments because the act of walking across campus may cause them to crash and prevent them from doing their job. These accessibility points remove uncertainty and fear related to living in their environment.

Complex chronic conditions have often been sidelined within disability consciousness, largely because these health problems are not inherently visible. In the case of a wheelchair user, they are irrevocably public with their disability because their access point to the world around them is through a visible tool. Many people who experience episodic disability, however, may experience periods of time when they are too exhausted to take a shower, make a meal, or dress, let alone leave their home. On some days, sunlight may pierce through their eyes and cause splitting headaches, requiring them to stay in a dark and quiet space until the raging pain subsides. Or they may have so much pain in their muscles and abdomen that moving around is impossible to conceive. On other days, however, they may be able to dress, work, shop, and move around in the world like they did before they got sick. For some, this type of activity may cause them to crash later, requiring days or weeks of rest to recover from a trip outside of their normal routine and effort.

But to the outsider, who may see their neighbor pushing a shopping cart at the local grocer, well dressed and cheerful, they might appear healthy and well. Krista Coombs, a long COVID patient activist and mother of children living with long COVID, said, "We all look okay. That's the problem. People don't see you when you're sick. They see when you're well. But they don't see the down days." An old family friend who once ran long distances quipped that this experience can be summed up as the "push and crash." He explained how you feel like you're getting back to normal, so you push too hard—you go for a walk, complete an extra errand, take on an extra shift or chore—and then you crash. For many, the crash is like a complete exhaustion where you can't sleep and you require days to recover enough to do routine things. For many people, the most difficult thing is gauging what they can and cannot do—and predicting when a crash will transpire. Yet, most people who don't experience this post-exertional malaise cannot understand why these people become so exhausted.

There is an important history to the marginalization of chronically ill people from the disability rights movements, in part because they were originally tethered to the League of the Physically Handicapped that was organized during the Great Depression. Civil rights laws like the Brown v Board of Education decision and the Civil Rights Act that ended school segregation cleared a path toward recognizing the rights of people with disabilities, as the 1973 Rehabilitation Act does. Legal scholar Doron Dorfman argues that the Americans with Disabilities Act broke "new ground in American legal tradition, not only by prohibiting disability discrimination in all areas of public life but also by further combining a distributive element of 'positive rights' that compels the state and private actors to affirmatively provide accommodations for disabled people."[3] However, this did not include all disabled people. Mobility-related physical disabilities were central to disability rights activists, like Judy Heumann, the mother of the disability rights movement, and they drove the writing of the Americans with Disabilities Act of 1990.

The disability justice movement, led by Black, brown, and queer folks, emerged at the turn of the century and offered an alternative framework to the long tradition of white, male, and mobility-centered activism embedded in the movement. This more-recent activism has led to several amendments to the original law, broadening the scope of what *disability* means and who is protected under the law.[4] For example, in one point of departure, the disability justice movement centered people with the most severe forms of disability, which included chronically ill people who may not immediately "look" sick.[5] In fact, the exclusion of chronically ill people from disability law has been a long-standing concern of the disability justice movement.[6]

Contemporary disability activism, which involves the concerns of chronically ill people, however, cannot be understood without tracing its roots to revolutionary front lines movements, such as global movements for Indigenous sovereignty, movements for racial justice in the United States, and movements of people with HIV and AIDS. In what follows, I describe how several "embodied health movements" transformed the landscape for chronically ill people to become central to disability movements. Sociologist Phil Brown and others use the term *embodied health movements* to describe how patients actively mobilize to demand recognition for "contested" conditions that are "either unexplained by current medical knowledge or have purported environmental explanations that are often disputed."[7]

FOUNDATIONS OF AIDS ACTIVISM

In the summer of 1982, news anchor Tom Brokaw hit the airwaves, reporting, "Scientists at the National Center for Disease Control in Atlanta today released the result of a study that shows that the lifestyle of some male homosexuals has triggered an epidemic of a rare form of cancer."[8] Illustrating how little was known at the time, reporter Robert Bazell emphasized that the condition made the body struggle to fight disease. Some, he explained, develop a rare cancer called Kaposi sarcoma, and others develop a type of pneumonia. The news report then shifted to an interview with Bobbi Campbell, a gay man, saying "I was in the fast lane at one time in terms of the way that I lived my life. And now I'm not." Bazell shored up the report, standing in front of the Center for Disease Control, and suggested that researchers believe "we are dealing with a new deadly sexually transmitted disease."[9]

This was less than a year after the CDC first published its *Morbidity and Mortality Weekly Report* noting that five young men in Los Angeles had been treated for a form of pneumonia. Two had died. The report observed the immunosuppression wrought by the condition, although the CDC mostly focused on the patients' sexuality. The CDC reported twenty-six cases a few weeks later, mostly in New York City but some in California, of young men with Kaposi sarcoma.[10] Kaposi sarcoma is a rare disease found mostly in the elderly that causes lesions to grow in the skin, lymph nodes, internal organs, and mucous lining of the mouth, nose, and throat. The cancer becomes visible as skin blotches that appear purple, red, or brown. The visibility of the cancers became frightening as the virus spread around the world.

The social stigma around HIV spun by these early media reports spread more quickly than the virus. While communities of gay men were increasingly blamed for the epidemic, a form of embodied patient activism emerged that transformed how patients engage with science, medicine, and government around emerging and complex health conditions. The patient activism in the early days of the AIDS epidemic, sociologist Steven Epstein argued in his book *Impure Science*, was unique in part because gay men became the face of HIV because a small community of well-connected and privileged patients were able to get access to private clinicians who took their condition seriously.[11]

Recognizing the role of these activists in elevating awareness for research and policy is critical and in great contrast to other groups unduly afflicted by HIV. For instance, in the same years, intravenous drug users, who reported similar levels of transmission, often died before getting adequate attention from the medical community.

What's remarkable about the HIV story is the flood of scientific and political attention it attracted, largely due to patient activism.[12] On the one hand, HIV was falsely understood as a problem of "GRID," or gay-related immune deficiency, a concept that influenced medical treatment during the early years of the AIDS pandemic.[13] On the other hand, contrasting narratives emerged that were often ignored in those early days. As early as 1983, there were several papers in *The Lancet*, a prominent British medical journal, suggesting that the condition could be associated with "immune overload" (while others were still stuck on homophobia, calling it the "promiscuity paradigm").[14] Patient activism responded to these pejorative frames by elevating the problems of what they called ironically "gay cancers" and "gay disease" to serve as a "rallying cry to alert gay men to the presence of a new danger" and to promote political action. This activism, according to Epstein, was also what made it remarkable.[15]

AIDS activists not only were patients but had multiple identities: reporters, doctors, policymakers, stockbrokers, teachers, and scientists. Gay reporters reported on HIV, often writing critically about medical and public health communities' tendency to "blame the epidemic on gay promiscuity."[16] Gay physicians were more likely to be sympathetic to the medical community but increasingly vocal about the condition. Epstein argued that "much as an earlier generation of feminists had conceived of medicine as a sexist institution, these writers and activists argued that medical science was a heterosexist and sexphobic institution that reinforced norms of sexual conformity."[17]

By 1987, AIDS activists had founded ACT UP, or the AIDS Coalition to Unleash Power, which was a protest organization that focused on elevating public action to fight the AIDS crisis. ACT UP was founded by Larry Kramer—a political organizer who witnessed firsthand the extraordinary pain and death from the crisis in the 1980s, which led him to co-found the Gay Men's Health Crisis (a private organization to support people living with AIDS). ACT UP fought for policy change and resources as well as to preserve people's own lives and health. They were not only on the "street" but also in NIH boardrooms, clinical spaces, and social gatherings, pushing for a broader and deeper agenda for HIV research and care.[18] ACT UP created strategies to assist people in seeking care when clinical contexts might be hostile or when clinicians might carry stigma, disbelief, or skepticism around a patient's symptoms or illness. For instance, they'd create four pages of notes with information to guide people in discussions about symptoms and illness with their doctors. These notes were printed on 11x17 paper so people could fold them up and put them in their pockets to be ready to advocate for themselves with their doctors.[19]

AIDS activism was rapid, organized, and strategic, enabling patient activists to cultivate an "alternative basis of expertise" that spoke truth to power in both medicine and politics.[20] They challenged government, engaged in deep dialogue with clinicians and medical establishments, grappled for power and relevance within and among advocates, found success in fundraising for research, and raised public awareness. In some cases, they literally laid their bodies on the line to raise awareness of their suffering. In doing so, ACT UP set a precedent for illness activism, proving to be a powerhouse for policy transformation and public awareness about the epidemic.[21] Yet, it's important to emphasize that ACT UP was central to AIDS activism in part because they had substantial financial and social resources as well as physical resources.[22]

The stigma and loss during this time, however, was devastating for many communities affected by the virus. At her dinner table in Atlanta, my aunt Cindy described to me how difficult it was to be a lesbian activist in the AIDS movement when her friends were dying from

AIDS. In the 1980s, she had a group of friends—mostly gay men—who she'd go out with to parties, bars, and clubs on the weekends. Over the course of a decade, every friend from that group died from AIDS. She was devastated, roiled by the depth of despair brought by the AIDS pandemic into her small circle of friends, and it was impossible to stay silent. Because so many men were dying in those earliest days, AIDS was long characterized as a male disease, and many women struggled to get diagnosed or treated. Early in the pandemic, a common mantra was "Women don't get AIDS; they just die from it." This mantra has relevance today when we think about a common long COVID mantra: "Long COVID's not real; it just destroys women's lives."

THE INVISIBILITY OF ME/CFS

When I first spoke to David Tuller, I realized that he had rubbed shoulders with Larry Kramer in the early days of the AIDS movement. As a young gay man in NYC in the 1980s, he worked in AIDS activism before ACT UP was officially formed. They marched on Washington, and Tuller was arrested twice, laying his body on the line to raise awareness that his friends were dying. He moved to San Francisco in 1988 for a job as a reporter at the *San Francisco Chronicle*. Although the newspaper's ethical guidelines prohibited him from joining advocacy organizations, he wrote extensively about HIV and AIDS activism for the *Chronicle*.

Tuller's passion for HIV activism expanded to ME/CFS when he moved from New York City to San Francisco, where he observed a community of sick people (mostly women). He was struck by the ways in which these patients were consistently marginalized in science and medicine at a time when people were throwing all their money and expertise behind the search for a cure for HIV. AIDS profoundly overshadowed the ME/CFS condition, in part because AIDS patients presented with visible lesions on their bodies and people were wasting away from the illness. At least in the eighties, those who got sick got sicker visibly fast and died. In contrast, Tuller noticed, those with ME/CFS would disappear into their private, internal worlds at home and become "invisible" to medicine, politics, and society. Although people don't usually die from ME/CFS, an estimated one in four people who had it were bedbound.[23] Tuller told me, "In HIV you can be super active until you're really sick. If you do that when you have ME, the more you do, the more you're going to get post-exertional malaise and get sicker."

Emily Lim Rogers, a medical anthropologist who writes about ME/CFS politics, has argued that one of the struggles for patient activists living with ME/CFS is that "activist movements also involve *movement*" and activism requires *action*.[24] Rogers described this struggle for visibility as the "dual-pronged challenge" of confronting "stigma caused by its lack of biological verification and societal acceptance" and protesting "in bodies that are exhausted."[25] Rogers has characterized this condition as a multifaceted feat of endurance where people living with ME/CFS must "endure" government neglect, living in sick bodies for which there is no treatment nor cure, and extraordinary "derision that comes with their disease."[26] This causes a sense of liminality where people are neither in crisis nor facing a death sentence (as with HIV and AIDS). Rather, they face an endurance of invisible illness.

The enduring nature of this condition causes many patients to lose steam for a visible life in activism, advocacy, or, in many cases, work. Billy Hanlon, ME activist and director of advocacy for the Minnesota ME/CFS Alliance, told me that many people he works with prefer to direct their efforts to nurturing their loved ones and their family lives, rather than pouring their limited energy into politics they don't think will change much. In doing so, people reorient their identities, social roles, and lives and redefine life priorities and meaning, in the face of an enduring illness with no treatment and no cure, to cultivate a meaningful life.

Other embodied health movements, like for breast cancer, have had more luck in part because they have had better evidence, learning the strategies from AIDS activists and using their "alternative basis of expertise" to demand attention, influence legislation, and raise funding for research and treatment.[27] Cancers became immensely more visible in part because they were verifiable conditions that were clearly identified within medical culture. Even still, the skills learned from AIDS activists played a vital role in political activism for breast cancer. A breast cancer activist explained how AIDS activists "showed us how to get through to the Government" and "took on an archaic system and turned it around while we have been quietly dying."[28]

In 1991, more than 180 US advocacy groups came together to form the National Breast Cancer Coalition. *The New York Times Sunday Magazine* wrote, "They say they've had it with politicians and physicians and scientists who 'there, there' them with studies and statistics and treatments that suggest the disease is under control."[29] Epstein explained how the coalition was, in their first year, able to convince Congress to increase funding for breast cancer research by $43 million, an increase of almost 50 percent. This amount was incomparable to the paucity of money attributed to ME/CFS and Lyme at the time. "The next year, armed with data from a seminar they financed, the women asked for, wheedled, negotiated and won a whopping $300 million more."[30]

Patient activism for ME/CFS emerged in the 1980s but remained limited in part because of the limitations of the health condition. The first record of a support group for ME/CFS was in 1985—just two years before ACT UP was founded, and one year after the discovery of HIV.[31] In 1987, Mark Iverson, a patient living with CFS, founded an organization called the CFIDS Association of America, using the early patient-defined term Chronic Fatigue and Immune Dysfunction Syndrome (CFIDS). For many years, this organization focused on fostering support within the patient community. In 1991, when Mark became too sick to run the group, Kim McCleary took over the reins and transformed the group to a patient activist group that focused on catalyzing research and transforming legislation. For instance, it was instrumental in developing a policy ruling for the Social Security Administration that recognized CFS as a disabling condition for the first time. Another example was through McCleary's appointment to a US advisory committee on chronic fatigue syndrome. This activism exposed the CDC's misuse of fundings to other health programs.[32] In 2014, the group changed its name to the Solve ME/CFS Initiative and has continued this strategic activism.

FLIPPING THE SCRIPT

In the past decade, how *sick women* speak truth to power has transformed largely through digital activism. For instance, Johanna Hedva, a disabled activist and scholar, provides an alternate way of thinking about the everyday lives and activism of disabled activists through their philosophical blogging about "Sick Woman Theory."[33] Hedva argues that the "private is political" in a way that pushes back against German historian and philosopher Hannah Arendt's contention that political action exists in "the public."[34] While Arendt's work moved the idea of political action from the hallowed walls of institutions and into the street, Hedva insists that many disabled people demonstrate activism in radically collective ways that are less visible than the ones Arendt suggested. Many disabled people avoid protests, not only because of mobility, but also due to legitimate fears of violence and the inaccessibility of spaces of protest. While these barriers make street protests difficult, it does not mean that those who remain home are *a*political. Instead, Hedva insists, "Most modes of political protest are internalized, lived, embodied, suffering, and therefore invisible."[35] In these ways, Hedva insists, protest may manifest in radical anti-capitalist actions of the everyday life with those you love (and those you do not love) through the "politics of care."[36] This involves caring for someone who is sick, or caring for yourself. It means working in historically feminized professions of caring in the most invisible ways through nursing, nurturing, and caring. It also involves the radical notion of recognizing people's "vulnerability and fragility and precarity" based on their positionality and power.[37]

As Hedva suggests, the private is political in the length of the showers you take, the number of likes you give to a social media post, and the GoFundMe sites people initiate to pay their escalating medical bills.[38] Digital activism for ME/CFS was activated in part by the founding of #MEAction. #MEAction is a patient activist organization devoted to elevating the online presence of ME through creative projects devoted to research, public education, and providing patients with support and knowledge. Jaime Seltzer, the science director of #MEAction, described how they have spent hundreds of hours developing content about history, concepts, and knowledge around ME/CFS to publish on #MEPedia, a public source of information that was built by patients, students, and researchers.[39] The #MEAction network was founded in 2015, around the same time Tuller started publishing about the PACE Trials. It was cofounded by Jennifer Brea, the Harvard PhD student who was disabled by ME, along with several other activists, including Seltzer. This activism has proven to be very influential in the ME/CFS space. In fact, Seltzer was named one of *TIME* magazine's one hundred most influential people in health in 2024.

#MEAction is an exemplar of what Lisa Diedrich calls hashtag activism, where illness- and disability-oriented hashtags on social media serve as "portals into the how and why illness and disability become *sites* of political struggle."[40] #MEAction, for example, has organized an annual protest since 2016 called #MillionsMissing, where they encourage people to "show up from home"—that is, send electronic messages—to elevate their goals to bring awareness to the needs of

ME/CFS patients in politics and medicine.[41] The first protest was organized in twelve locations, with pairs of shoes placed a foot apart to mark how many people have lost their social lives and ability to physically protest, due to their illness. In 2024, I participated in a #MEAction (Maryland chapter) protest at Georgetown University where we placed empty cots at the center of campus to demonstrate the millions of bedbound patients. Each year, the organizers have a particular objective: in 2016, it was to increase research funding and clinical trials for ME/CFS. In 2024, it was to elevate medical education through targeted partnerships in a campaign called #TeachMETreatME.[42] These forms of hashtag activism elevate political movements through digital spaces; then they become points of access for disabled activists around the world.

AN EMBODIED ACTIVIST

I wanted to learn more about the lived experience of this activism, so I reached out to disability activist JD Davids on a sunny afternoon in mid-October. JD identifies as a 55-year-old disabled, white, queer, and trans person of Ashkenazi Jewish descent, living with ME/CFS and several other complex chronic conditions, including long COVID. As a young person, JD was constantly sick with viral and bacterial infections, compounded by allergies that were constantly acting up. JD's immune system was too weak in some ways and overactive in others. Missing school and feeling different from his classmates amplified his fear of judgment among his peers. This was in part because he was one of few Jewish kids in his community and was puzzled by common gendered expectations.

A decade into the AIDS pandemic, JD finished college and started volunteering with ACT UP. Joining this collective of activists was transformative for him as he began to understand his own queerness where "illness was the norm, not the exception."[43] In this way, JD felt accepted and whole amongst a crew of sick people and allies, queer people, people who use drugs—former and current—and others committed to working, in his words, to "save ourselves, our loved ones, our friends."[44] It was exactly this diversity of activists, and complexity of needs and priorities that made AIDS activism so complicated, vibrant, and effective.

JD explained how lesbian activism in ACT UP in Philadelphia and elsewhere stemmed in part from the women's movement. Women literally had to take matters into their own hands, as JD wrote, "using speculums and flashlights to learn what their cervixes looked like, while at the same time critiquing how medical establishments talked about gender, women, reproduction, and sex."[45] This embodied health activism set a strong precedence for what power communities could collectively garner to create an inclusive environment and fight against the medical establishment that they felt did not hear them or understand their needs.

It was the HIV community where JD learned how to advocate for his own health, which would become essential in his activism for people with ME/CFS and long COVID later. JD described how most people with ME don't have a diagnosis, which is one of the reasons they don't have treatment or care. Yet, what is challenging, JD explained, is that many forms of immune suppression or immune alteration change how people live. "But they don't die from it," he explained, comparing both ME/CFS and long COVID activists with ACT UP activists from the early days of the pandemic. This was particularly concerning when COVID-19 emerged and "people were talking about us but not to us, and people were already talking about how COVID wasn't a problem because it would affect people who were already sick or disabled." JD and others organized a webinar then—in March 2020—for chronically ill people to prepare them to deal with the pandemic.

JD explained that part of the uphill battle faced by people living with ME/CFS and long COVID is a cultural bias against those who are chronically ill. "There is such deep bias, stigma, and honestly hatred of sick people," JD explained. "People not only do not want to acknowledge it until it inherently happens to them, or even sometimes it has happened to them. It still doesn't change it. But also, so many forces are telling them that's not happening. And people will say, 'If there was this many people with long COVID, I would know people.' And it harkens back to the metaphor that there's plenty of people who don't think they know trans people, or there used to be people who thought they didn't know gay people, like, that's not the point. But that's people's deep-seated denial, that they're being encouraged to have this denial. Even when people are sick, become sick, or become disabled, what we're supposed to do is put all of our hopes and efforts into things called cures, or becoming unsick or undisabled, instead of having the support to have lives with dignity and ease, no matter what our current bodily status is."

Bringing these patients out of the shadows is essential because so often others do not believe that they are sick. People who are already immunocompromised because of ME/CFS or HIV were already dealing with "a lot of stigma about disability and illness," JD commented. He said, "The associations of lack of worth, of shame, and then of the realistic fears of economic and social marginalization if someone is sick or disabled, are huge." I nodded, thinking about the ways in which HIV opened a conversation about episodic disability, where people came to recognize how an illness ebbs and flows from one day to the next.[46]

By amplifying the possibility of doing activism from one's bed, as Emily Lim Rogers and Johanna Hedva have written about, disability justice activists have provided a powerful rethink of what disability justice looks like and how people living with unpredictable physical bodies, who experience episodic or dynamic disability, may still engage in important advocacy.[47] Disability activist, anthropologist, and theologian Erin Raffety has suggested that despite "creative and online forms of resistance" and a "broad, intersectional definition of disability [that] has been somewhat more inclusive to chronically ill people, especially during the COVID-19 pandemic, disjunctures between chronically ill people and disability rights movements persist."[48]

On the one hand, the concept of disability can be difficult for chronically ill people, in part because it cultivates an unease about the permanence of their condition. Dorfman told me, "A struggle for long COVID is for people to be identified as disabled. People are reluctant to be called disabled because a person's identity really affects how they see themselves and interact with the law. There are procedures for them to gain legal protections or legal benefits." He went on to explain, "I think there is reluctance from long COVID patients to consider themselves disabled, or to consider that their conditions are not temporary."[49] Relatedly, Dorfman and others have described disability-related stigma as the stated or implied accusation that they are running a "disability con"; that is, people who use disability accommodations feel others question their disability, especially when it may be less visible, making people look "suspicious."[50] This is particularly true for people who experience dynamic disability, or the disability that ebbs and flows with chronic illness that was coined "episodic disability" by people living with HIV.[51] JD explained how difficult these perceptions are in professional circles, where "it doesn't necessarily mean that we're going to be able to afford to acknowledge that we have an illness or a disability. Because under sort of a capitalist mindset, [people make us feel that] we're not worthy unless we're productive."

Yet, long COVID patient activism may be at a turning point. In the last decade, the surge of interest in online support groups and collective organizing has ballooned so much that there is not enough admin capacity to provide patients with a platform. The sheer interest among people living with dynamic disabilities eager to amplify the need for a more dynamic way of thinking about disability underscores the need for a cultural shift in how disability is perceived and enacted in American culture.

LONG COVID ACTIVISM

In May 2020, Italian archaeologist Elisa Perego, living with disabling symptoms in the wake of an acute SARS-CoV-2 infection, first tweeted the hashtag #LongCovid on Twitter (now X). She was residing in the region of Lombardy in northern Italy, an early epicenter of the pandemic, where many people suffered not only from the acute virus but also from a constellation of lingering symptoms. Describing her personal journey with the condition as cyclical, progressive, and multiphasic, Perego attracted thousands of retweets.[52]

Around the same time, Fiona Lowenstein was already using digital activism to bring together other people exhibiting chronically severe and disabling symptoms following an acute bout of virus. Lowenstein explained in *The New York Times*, "I felt alone in my healing process. I wanted information, and to connect with others who shared my experience."[53] At the beginning of the pandemic, Lowenstein was the president of a queer feminist wellness collective called Body Politic that, rooted in the disability justice movement, cultivated a space for inclusivity, accessibility, and crucial discussions about health, well-being, and justice.[54] Lowenstein and Body Politic board member Sabrina Bleich initiated an online support group in WhatsApp for people suffering from long COVID that grew to help more than fourteen thousand members residing in over thirty countries.[55] Many people sought these communities because in 2020 they, like Lowenstein, felt completely alone: they felt dismissed and disbelieved by family, friends, and clinicians.

Supported early on by multiple disability rights groups, Body Politic activists connected long COVID patients with resources, information, and communities, quickly mobilizing a movement that became a source of comfort, information, and companionship for an illness that many people would not formally recognize for some time. For many people living with long COVID, this was the only space in their life where they felt comfortable sharing their experience and where others believed that their symptoms were real. Body Politic eventually transferred the WhatsApp group to Slack, where several channels formed, fostering distinct patient communities. Two channels of note developed into independent research and advocacy groups. One is known as Long Covid SOS, a UK-based charity that focuses on elevating knowledge and awareness of long COVID through the recognition of, research on, and rehabilitation among those living with long COVID. Another Slack channel known as "data nerds" became an independent organization known as the Patient-Led Research Collaboration, or PLRC.

PLRC was motivated to "study ourselves" because they felt so dismissed by clinicians and in medical settings.[56] The PLRC was formed when Hanna Davis, Lisa McCorkell, Gina Assaf, Hannah Wei, and Athena Akrami organized a survey—despite being very sick from long COVID—to systematically document their symptoms and build the first patient-led database of long COVID symptoms.[57] They published the first survey and research report of people with long COVID in an open Google Doc and eventually published it in The Lancet's *eClincial-Medicine* journal.[58] They then conducted a follow-up survey with more than two hundred symptoms, including write-in symptoms from the first survey (like post-exertional malaise, tremors, tinnitus, heart palpitations), as well as social issues like one's ability to work. They also developed other programs that prioritized patient concerns, needs, and perspectives.[59] For instance, patients served as a review panel for determining what research projects should be funded. They then founded a journal called *Patient-Generated Hypotheses*, a novel and pathbreaking journal for medical science, prioritizing the ideas and projects of scientists and funders living with long COVID.[60]

Although the Body Politic Slack groups shut down due to lack of funding, their ongoing digital presence promotes other ground-up patient-led groups devoted to elevating the health and well-being of long COVID patients. For instance, they work closely with Karyn Bishop, a single mom who launched the COVID-19 Longhauler Advocacy Project in June 2020.[61] After Bishop got sick, she lost her job as an emergency responder and was too disabled to go back to work. She dove into collecting surveys and polls of the long COVID community to use for advocacy. The COVID-19 Longhauler Advocacy Project founded a chapter in every state, and a few other chapters focused on special populations like caretakers, partners, and support circles. This ground-up research serves to raise awareness with the federal government to advocate for better medical coverage and disability insurance for long-haulers. Other organizations include The Mighty (a nonmedia platform for peer support), #MEAction, Bateman Horne Center (for zoom support meetings), and several private Facebook groups, such as Dysautonomia International, Black COVID-19 Survivors, Long Covid Support, and Long Covid Families.

Journalist Ryan Prior chronicled work by Lowenstein, Perego, and others in *The Long Haul: How Long Covid Survivors Are Revolutionizing Healthcare*. He described how activist women used the energy they did have—despite being very sick from long COVID—to organize online and change the face of the pandemic. Referring to these activists, Ziyad Al-Aly, a clinician, epidemiologist, and professor of medicine at Washington University in St. Louis, said, "It's really possible that they changed the history of medicine."[62]

While patient activism has largely been patient focused, the urgency around patient activism has bolstered rapid scientific discovery for long COVID. Much of this research has built upon decades of previous research about ME/CFS and other complex chronic conditions, from lupus to Lyme disease. Scientists have identified several pathways through which COVID-19 causes long-term dysregulation of the body via the blood, brain, gut, and other tissues. Much of this research was going on long before SARS-CoV-2 emerged, although it was somewhat marginalized, considered obscure, and underfunded. For example,

Harvard neuroscience researcher Michael VanElzakker and microbiologist Amy Proal together founded the nonprofit PolyBio Research Foundation, which was designed to focus on understanding how postviral conditions make people sick and why. Since long COVID rose to prominence, PolyBio has risen in notoriety and research dollars. Their work—informed by a decade of theoretical thinking—has been influential for understanding long COVID biology, theorizing where the virus hides and what it does to dysregulate multiple systems.[63]

Even still, clinician skepticism remains strong in some contexts and has dissipated in others. Many physicians have contracted long COVID themselves, serving as powerful patient activists. Innovators in medicine, such as David Putrino, the director of rehabilitation innovation at Mount Sinai Health System in New York, have had a measurable impact on revolutionizing how clinical care is designed and delivered for people living with long COVID. Putrino described to Prior how, like others in embodied health movements, he has been motivated by "a core guiding principle of community co-design" and a "nothing about us without us" mentality.[64] This framing harkens back to the earliest AIDS activists as well as activists from the disability justice movement and mental health advocates. These practitioners are translating knowledge of long COVID patients to a broader medical audience and encouraging a deep rethink about how we care for patients living with complex chronic conditions in medical settings, which tend to focus on a specific organ, function, or area of the body to diagnose and treat.

Hashtag activism has also become an important conduit of science education, in some cases connecting a curious public directly with cutting-edge scientists, as well as shifting the narrative about whose stories matter. For example, Akiko Iwasaki, an immunobiologist at Yale, transformed the COVID landscape by educating people on Twitter (now X) and sharing extensive content about what was known and unknown about long COVID symptoms. This work had an extraordinary impact on Iwasaki's own understanding of the virus, contributing to medical innovations, such as administering a nasal COVID-19 vaccine.[65] Hashtag activism has also affected how society perceives conditions like ME/CFS and long COVID. Patient activists have fought to recognize the complex faces of long COVID, bringing intersectional differences of patients out of the shadows. For instance, Imani Barbarin's advocacy through #MyDisabledLifeIsWorthy inspired thousands of disabled people to engage in public debates around long COVID.[66] Similarly, Chimére Sweeney has elevated the experience of Black long COVID storytellers by promoting the production of the documentary #BlackandUnBelieved film.[67] Her activism has been influential in demanding that Black women are featured in stories about long COVID, and that long COVID advocacy spaces are more inclusive.[68]

These efforts continue to receive attention in part because so many people are living with long COVID without a diagnosis, treatment, and disability accommodations. The last factor remains an urgent matter for many long COVID patients because they can no longer work, many have lost their homes, some have lost their social networks, and many people who developed long COVID at the beginning of the COVID-19 pandemic continue to experience persistent symptoms. For some, the need for disability accommodations has become a matter of life and death, and legal counsel has become one of the most essential health interventions.

Like many embodied health movements, from breast cancer awareness to the AIDS movement, the global long COVID activist movement reveals its power by building community locally, nationally, and globally. In some ways, this is what makes long COVID unique—an extraordinary pandemic swept across the globe and left lingering effects on people in different cultures, political contexts, and health systems. Together, patient activists have been able to share information to challenge governments, engage in deep dialogue with clinicians and medical establishments, fundraise for research, and raise public awareness. While there were often hints of small moves where patient activists grappled for power and relevance within and among advocates (demonstrated by the global proliferation of advocacy groups, which sometimes involves infighting), the patient community has proven to be unlike other patient movements, in part because of the extraordinarily vast impacts of digital activism.

7

STRUCTURAL SILENCING

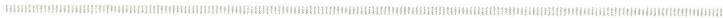

IN SOME WAYS, Ty Godwin was lucky. He'd been married for years to a loving partner before he got sick. He'd worked as a business executive and had plenty of savings. He owned his home. When he got sick, he received disability from his company and quickly qualified for Social Security Disability. At first, Ty had good medical coverage. And he had an appetite for the recovery journey, spending hours researching tests, treatments, and possible solutions.

Ty is a white business executive in his midfifties who lost his career and his identity as a marathon runner to long COVID. When he lost his ability to compete in marathons, Ty committed his energy to searching for answers to explain his deteriorating health. Ty's appetite for answers, however, was expensive, and he often overextended his medical premiums. I asked Ty to estimate what his medical expenses were over the past several years. I was curious about how much you might spend searching for answers if you could. I also knew Ty was generous and willing to share his journey, because he wrote about some of these experiences on his blog.[1]

Since 2020, Ty's costs have varied from year to year. He estimates that during the first 3.5 years of living with long COVID, he spent nearly $30,000 on medical expenses. He also spent around $61,000 on medical premiums, which escalated when he had to move to COBRA. COBRA is a program that enables someone out of work to maintain their health insurance from a previous job; however, it requires that person to cover both the part they had paid and what their employer had paid previously. In addition, Ty spent another $18,000 out of pocket to travel to the Mayo Clinic and to Martinos Center for Biomedical Imaging at Massachusetts General Hospital to seek answers from experts. Along the way, he spent another $11,000 on alternative therapies, including neurofeedback mapping and therapy. He also spent more than $3,000 on additional testing to better understand his biology, including a test that proved his mitochondria were damaged. This is a common problem among people struggling with disabling fatigue—but there isn't an effective therapy for it, and it's not clear what the root cause of the mitochondrial damage might be.

Ty's affluence puts him in the category of the sick elite. Yet, Ty lost more than a million dollars in wages after he got sick. And, unfortunately, in 2024, Ty was diagnosed with stage 4 cancer. His oncologist theorized that COVID-19 damaged his immune system and could have contributed to or exacerbated his cancer. Yet, unlike with long COVID—where insurance coverage is not always reliable—most of Ty's cancer treatment was covered by Medicare and his supplemental health insurance (paid out of pocket). In this case, Ty's cancer was a verifiable health condition with medications that were available to treat what ailed him. He is not out of the woods, however, and continues to wade through the murky waters of illness.

Few people I spoke to were like Ty, however. Instead, many people shared an experience more akin to that of a grandmother I'll call Theresa. Theresa is an elderly white woman who was living on a shoestring budget in Alabama. She drove a local bus for 24 years. But then her husband died, and she needed more money. She found a new job at the casino in town right before everything shut down. That's where she got COVID-19 for the first time. At first, she wasn't too sick. But then she got it again. Then again. And again. She had gotten sicker with each infection, and the symptoms wouldn't go away. Her energy dropped, her weight spiked, and her world got very small. She saved all the energy she did have to care for her granddaughter and to generate the energy to head to the clinic for medical care.

For years, Theresa had a doctor she trusted. He cared for her through pregnancy, parenting, and aging—he was someone she had always relied on, and her husband's health insurance ensured she could keep seeing him. She was able to maintain her insurance when she took the job at the casino. But when she lost that job because she was so sick after COVID, she also lost her health insurance. Unfortunately, her doctor of 30 years did not accept Medicaid patients, so she had to seek care elsewhere. She told me she was counting down the days until she was eligible for Medicare so she could go back to the doctor she adores. Even more, Theresa worried that her new doctors were prescribing her too many medications, and she wondered if they were doing any good.[2] Since becoming ill, Theresa went from taking four medications per day to taking twenty. Still, the new clinicians would not diagnose her with long COVID.

Theresa had a strong family network and supportive community. However, she felt she did not have the finances to advocate for better health care. She couldn't qualify for Medicare because she wasn't 65, and her disability application had yet to be approved. She knew she had to work with these new doctors, but she worried about asking her new doctors *why* she was taking so many medications and not feeling better. And, why didn't she have a diagnosis? In many ways, Theresa felt she was silenced by the limitations of Medicaid, while she waited to qualify for Medicare so she could return to the doctor she trusted.

Inequity in the US health system makes it nearly impossible for people living with unverifiable health conditions to get the care they need, particularly if they rely on limited or unreliable medical insurance coverage.[3] While patients need to know they are believed, they cannot heal well without reliable health insurance that does not break the bank and cherry-pick what treatments are covered, defining some as *medically* necessity and not others. Even though an elite minority of people may do well with private health insurance or paying out of pocket for health care (like Ty), most people struggle because of this systemic inequality (like Theresa). Part of this problem is the limited public options we have for health care in America. And it's worse for people who had precarious health care coverage before getting sick, causing millions of Americans to fall into medical bankruptcy.

Many people like Theresa turn to crowdfunding to cover their medical costs. The moral economies of crowdfunding, however, play a profound role in *who* gets funded and *how much* they raise. In her groundbreaking book *Crowded Out*, medical anthropologist Nora Kenworthy argues that the idea of crowdfunding itself is a very American idea, not only because our health system is broken, but also for cultural reasons.[4] Crowdfunding is advertised as a "marketplace of equal opportunity" that gives everyone a strong footing to overcome whatever struggle they face. Yet, the pressure people feel to edit their stories comes from "highly competitive economies like GoFundMe," and there is little room for "human fallibility here, nor for those who struggle . . . with chronic health conditions that often elicit blame or assumptions that one's ill health is due to individual behaviors or decisions."[5] In this way, even digital options can be limited when people struggle with conditions the public might not understand.

STRUCTURAL SILENCING

Jodi Roque is a Spanish-speaking family physician who works at a federally qualified health clinic on the southwest side of Chicago. Most of her patients are uninsured, and many are undocumented. I've known Roque for years. We were chemistry partners in college, and on weeknights we volunteered as translators for Spanish-speaking patients seeking medical care at a local free clinic. I reached out to her to learn more about how she was caring for patients who came into her clinic with unexplainable symptoms that appeared untreatable. Roque made it clear that biomedicine wasn't the only barrier to untangling the knot of sickness people brought with them into the clinic. At the end of the day, she explained, it's about money—or the financial arrangements that make it so expensive and difficult to access medical care in America.

Roque described how every day at work is an absolute scramble. Because her patients are largely uninsured, she tries to order only the tests the clinic will cover. She is consistently overbooked and forced to work at a frantic, overwhelmingly fast pace to provide care to the vulnerable populations she serves. She said, "Unfortunately, a lot of my patients, even when I might refer them for additional tests, are not able to go. For example, I don't know if my patients truly have asthma because they cannot go for appropriate pulmonary function testing."

This is a classic case of structural vulnerability—when the systems and laws in place create barriers to resources and decision-making for people in desperate need of reliable and routine medical care.[6] "It's just hard to advocate for specialists for people without insurance," Roque said with a sigh and a shake of the head. "We apply for charity care, but it's hard to get, and care is often delayed. So, my ability to do additional workup and testing for uninsured patients with symptoms of long COVID is often pretty limited. Oftentimes, I do basic labs, try inhalers, help people quit smoking and so on, but there is not a lot that I can do other than just listen to them, believe and support them, and give them time to heal."

Recognizing these structural impediments to living well is a common thread in medical anthropology. Seth Holmes, a medical anthropologist and physician, argued that such challenges result when the "pressures of the current neoliberal capitalist system of health care and its financing force health professionals into a double bind. Either they spend the time and energy necessary to listen to and fully treat the patient and put their job and clinic in economic jeopardy, or they move at a frenetic pace to keep their practice afloat and only partially attend to the patient in their presence."[7]

Building on this way of thinking, I argue that people living with complex chronic conditions who face structural vulnerabilities in their health and well-being also experience a form of structural silencing. The silencing comes from the dismissal of complex and difficult-to-verify symptoms because clinicians are overworked, stressed, distracted, and rushed. In some cases, this might be outright gaslighting. In other cases, it might be a case of overt exhaustion and lack of understanding. While these forms of structural vulnerability are implicit, the lack of knowledge about complex chronic conditions is part of the larger structural silencing in medical training, where few hours are devoted to understanding ME/CFS, fibromyalgia, autoimmune conditions, and other systemic mysteries. In addition to what's typically perceived as structural *vulnerability* or *violence* is this silencing by withholding a rigorous and robust generation of knowledge and training around recognizing and caring for people living with unverifiable health conditions.

This was the case for Ja'Mia Hewitt, who had a difficult time getting a diagnosis even though she was constantly becoming dizzy and blacking out during her childhood. Eventually, she sought a career in nursing to better understand what was disrupting her health so frequently. For Ja'Mia, structural silencing began at the age of eight when she passed out for the first time while her mom was giving her a haircut. In her first clinical encounter, where she was told there was nothing wrong, suspicion crept in. Throughout her childhood, she continued to experience dizziness and would occasionally black out because she didn't understand what triggered her episodes. It wasn't until she was nineteen that her doctors tested her for postural orthostatic tachycardia syndrome (POTS), a form of dysautonomia. POTS makes your heart race, blood pressure spike, and breathing become labored. The doctors gave her the tilt table test, where you lie on a rotating table hooked up to machines to monitor your heart and blood pressure. They see if your blood pressure and heart rate respond to different positions, as you are moved quickly from lying down to sitting or standing. Ja'Mia's blood pressure raced, and she passed out. Yet, her doctor said everything looked fine. Years later, when she was pregnant with her first child, a doctor revisited her results and was baffled that she had never been diagnosed with POTS. Given the unequivocal diagnosis, the first clinician who reviewed Ja'Mia's exam could have been rushed, uncertain, uncomfortable, or unfamiliar with POTS, engaged in a form of structural silencing.

Ja'Mia's frustration with her experience as a patient led her to study nursing. "I'm like, enough is enough. I'm going to do whatever I can do to help ensure other people don't have to deal with what I'm dealing with." She told me, "Navigating this health care system is like pulling teeth." Part of her determination to understand the health system was due to her experience of such clear discrimination as a Black woman. Ja'Mia said, "Racism is alive and well in the US." In fact, her nursing skills probably saved her life: when she became sick with long COVID, she navigated her way through the Cleveland Clinic, where she was diagnosed with small fiber neuropathy, POTS, fibromyalgia, Sjögren's syndrome, sleep apnea, and long COVID.

In many ways, Ja'Mia's situation is a best-case scenario. First, she is aware of her body, her rights, and her needs. When things felt wrong, she sought care, was believed, and was sent to a specialty clinic where she was diagnosed for "illnesses you have to fight to get."[8] Even though her care was completely disorganized and dysfunctional, she has an educational background and experience to navigate a fragmented medical system and get the care she needed. However, for so many people in the United States, feeling dismissed or silenced during clinical encounters fuels an extraordinary amount of mistrust, particularly among Black Americans.[9] While complex chronic conditions are largely ignored and dismissed across the medical system, particularly when they are unverified, it's much worse for patients who are already marginalized due to intersectional identities within a difficult-to-navigate medical system.

ENACTING MISTRUST

Most people I spoke to described how they felt when a clinician told them that they did not believe that they were sick. What's important to realize is that everyone had their own story—and spoke their own truth. In what follows, I consider a form of structural silencing that relays how engagements with the medical system make people question their own perception of reality. Central to this way of thinking is Miranda Fricker's concept of epistemic injustice, which homes in on "wrong done to someone specifically in their capacity as a knower."[10]

Fricker divides forms of social power into two levels. On the one hand, there is hermeneutical injustice, when a gap in resources and power (such as between a patient and clinician) puts someone at an unfair disadvantage when it comes to making sense of their personal experiences. Fricker gives experiencing sexual harassment in a culture that lacks that critical concept as an example.[11] This gap applies directly to structural silencing because few clinicians have been trained to recognize, diagnose, and treat people with complex chronic health conditions, thereby rendering those patients' experiences and bodies invisible. This is particularly salient for a "new" health condition like long COVID for which people have not cultivated a shared language to convey what they are going through, thereby undermining their "authority".[12]

On the other hand, testimonial injustice speaks to the moment in a clinical encounter when a person in power (such as a clinician), which Fricker calls "the hearer," deflates the credibility of the speaker's word. Fricker gives the example of a police officer not believing someone because they are Black. This translates well to clinical encounters, where many people describe how multiple levels of their identity play a powerful role in the "credibility economy." In this case, a clinician would have "a credibility excess"—where a clinician might hold more power in a clinical interaction because of their medical degree, even if they have had limited exposure to complex chronic health conditions. Even still, sexism, racism, classism, and ableism are some of the forms of bias that likely influences the power dynamics between patient and clinician. At the same time, a patient might have "a credibility deficit" simply because of their identity as a patient, even if they are a medical doctor themselves.[13] As Fricker argues, "prejudice will tend surreptitiously to inflate or deflate the credibility afforded the speaker, and sometimes this will be sufficient to cross the threshold for belief or acceptance so that the hearer's prejudice causes him to miss out on a piece of knowledge."[14]

This brings us back to structural silencing. When an overburdened clinician is asked questions that they cannot answer, they must do their best to answer them, particularly if a patient has waited weeks or months for an appointment. This situation is complicated because a patient *assumes* that the clinician can properly identify, diagnose, and treat what ails them. Fricker suggests that what goes wrong often is an ethical dilemma for the clinician when "any attempts to disabuse them of their inflated view of his expertise would damage the doctor-patient relationship by unduly undermining their confidence in him" even if "he is aware that his best advice might yet mislead them about an important health issue."[15] This puts a clinician in a double bind, where they may feel they must use the power they do have to put the patient at ease, even when they might feel powerless to act.

ANTI-BLACKNESS AND COMPLEX CHRONIC
HEALTH CONDITIONS

The credibility economy creates an undue burden on patients living with complex chronic conditions, and particularly on Black women patients. Oni Blackstock, a physician, Black woman, and health justice movement leader, spoke with me about how Black women face extraordinary levels of distrust and disbelief when they seek care, particularly for chronic pain and other unverifiable conditions. Blackstock said, "Why is white women's fatigue taken seriously but not Black women's fatigue taken seriously?" In our conversation Blackstock asked: Why are complex chronic conditions so commonly reported and amplified for white women (as well as white men) while we have evidence that Black and brown people are experiencing the same or worse symptoms? Blackstock explained that it's being a person of color and being a woman—"It's a double whammy of not getting care." In this way, intersectionality, or the multiple forms of identity that lead to discrimination and injustice, plays an essential role in the credibility economy.[16] For Black and brown women experiencing a chronic health condition—a state of being that is already at odds within our medical system—getting access to adequate care is much harder.

Blackstock explained how even she—a well-respected physician—often informs a new provider that she too is a physician, because she expects to be treated poorly. In this case, Blackstock employs a power lever to enhance her credibility within that clinical space, in anticipation of testimonial injustice. This is not an unfounded bias—it is based on years of experience.[17] When she brought this experience to Twitter (now X)—saying she did this because she wants the doctor to realize "I know what's going on here, or the way to protect myself"—a huge response flooded her feed from Black women-presenting physicians who do the same. She went on, "I think folks from minoritized groups are familiar with not having their concerns taken seriously. And I think typically when there's something vague like chronic fatigue syndrome, things are more unclear . . . it has to do with the biomedical model . . . when we can't put something into a clear bucket or category or can't provide some explanation for whatever we're seeing in terms of manifestations, physicians tend to struggle."

When complex chronic health conditions meet anti-Black bias in medicine, patients suffer. Anthropologist Chelsey Carter's work charts how Black and brown patients who have the rare disease amyotrophic lateral sclerosis (ALS) struggle to get a diagnosis because of a common belief among physicians that ALS is a "white disease." ALS is a progressive neurodegenerative disease that attacks the brain and spinal cord, weakens the muscles, and eventually causes paralysis and death within five years of the onset of symptoms. Little is known about risk and disease pathogenesis, but we do know that most ALS cases are sporadic, although some researchers have linked about 10 percent of cases to genes and biomarkers.[18] This small subset of patients carrying these biomarkers are all white.[19] Some researchers believe they hold the key to unlocking the mysteries of the disease, and an extraordinary amount of funding and research is focused solely on this population. This sits in stark contrast to Black people living with ALS, who are often misdiagnosed and excluded from clinical research trials because, Carter says, "researchers refused to consider that Black patients are afflicted with ALS."[20]

The unique experience of structural silencing among people of color living with complex chronic conditions is something Chelsey Carter describes with the term *neuroracism*. Carter defines neuroracism by the fact that white people's ALS stories are "foregrounded in public imaginations of ALS, and diagnostic biases based on race and gender negatively impact the lived experiences of Black people with ALS."[21] By perpetuating a biological narrative that ALS is a white disease, they subsequently deny Black people care, despite their symptoms and illness progression. Carter's work documents how medical racism, particularly in neurology and neuroscience, exists in cycles of diagnostic lapses, race-based diagnoses, health omissions, anti-Black gaslighting, and dismissive and negligent doctor-patient interactions.[22]

The concept of neuroracism can also inform how we understand systemic lupus erythematosus (SLE), a chronic autoimmune disease, which is sometimes considered a "Black" disease. Lupus is a verifiable disease that is characterized by an irregular autoimmune response where someone's body attacks their healthy cells, causing inflammation and destabilizing the kidneys, heart, and nervous system. Much like other complex chronic conditions characterized by dysautonomia, nine in ten people diagnosed with lupus are women. Yet, Black and brown women tend to develop lupus at an earlier age and have more severe and progressive illness than white women.[23] This is not only due to everyday weathering associated with stresses from employment, housing, and living with a debilitating illness; it also represents a classic case of structural silencing, where discrimination in medical settings, often in the form of being overlooked, dismissed, or outright disbelieved, causes these delays and afflictions.[24]

Carter's framework of neuroracism may apply to lupus in part because, as medical anthropologist Sandra Lane told me, some Black women are diagnosed with lupus when they have *any* symptoms of autoimmune diseases, even though their condition might not be lupus. Many women of color are not diagnosed at all, or their diagnoses are overshadowed by more common primary diagnoses. American writer Imani Barbarin has written about how Black disabled people in particular experience more misdiagnoses due to "culturally insensitive medical education."[25] In this case, lupus may be viewed as a "Black" disease because there is some biological risk for the autoimmune condition. Another possibility is that lupus exemplifies how race-based medicine reinforces an assumption that Black women presenting with symptoms of dysautonomia, or any of the cross-linked conditions discussed in this book, have lupus. Instead, they could have a smattering of other possible cross-linked conditions that present like lupus. When race is used in medical decision-making, it blurs the reality that someone may be experiencing, because bias fogs medical imagination. This is where structural silencing again may reflect the limited training clinicians have around complex chronic conditions, combined with neuroracism around the condition of lupus, driving up diagnoses and complicating treatments, possibly contributing to the high rates of late diagnosis or misdiagnosis.

WHEN CARE HARMS

In the mid-1990s, Kendra Hatfield-Timajchy was one of the first ethnographers to document the lives of women living with lupus.[26] Kendra met Marian—a middle-class single Black woman whose life had unraveled from lupus—in a support group in Atlanta. By the time they met, Marian's symptoms had brought her on an exhaustive diagnostic odyssey to seven physicians in the fields of primary care, endocrinology, infectious disease, neurology, and rheumatology over the span of two years.[27] The support group was exclusively for Black women, although they permitted Kendra, a white woman, to participate as an observer.

Kendra became close to Marian and four other women in the support group, attending the group meetings and often visiting them in their homes and accompanying them to medical appointments. Kendra and Marian became particularly close, and when Marian's health quickly deteriorated, she needed a strong social and family network to support her. She'd lost her job, health, and social network, and she was barely surviving on disability. The support group had become a sustaining presence in her life, and given Kendra's health and interest in lupus, she became a support system for Marian.

Kendra found, over time, that there was a single rheumatologist who Marian and the other women were seeing in Atlanta. And, over time, she realized something unusual was going on. Looking back,

Kendra wishes she had questioned the doctor's authority to continue drugs that were making Marian visibly sick. Kendra worried that he was "experimenting with various chemotherapies" that made her sicker. She realized after months of observation that a certain drug might be causing Marian's demise.

Although the doctor used the drug with many of his most severe patients, Kendra worried that the women she knew from the support group were becoming incredibly ill. She quickly moved from researcher to advocate because the women she was shadowing needed help, and they didn't know where to get it. Some had sisters or brothers, or parents, who could step in and advocate for them. Kendra explained, "What I observed very clearly was that in a crisis situation, you absolutely have to have someone with you in the room checking the medications and the dosages that they're giving you. You know the nurses mean well, but they're completely overwhelmed, or the doctors write an order that somehow gets mistranslated into their patient record. Having someone negotiating that and to basically protect you and lobby for you in that situation is critical."

Advocacy amidst structural silencing—when you are ignored or dismissed for your disability, race, ethnicity, gender, nationality, or age—is a crucial element of navigating illnesses that are hard to see and difficult to treat. In this situation, advocacy changes the power dynamic within testimonial injustice because there is a third party to weigh in, thereby tipping the scales. Unfortunately, it was too late for Marian. She only lived two more years after she met Kendra.

Women approaching menopause, like Marian, often experience misdiagnosis because some symptoms associated with menopause may overlap with, be intensified by, and weave together with other conditions, from endometriosis and dysautonomia to fibromyalgia and lupus. This was the experience of Chimére L. Sweeney—a schoolteacher turned long COVID activist—who struggled for two years to get someone to believe she was sick. The pain that shot through her neck and curved around her head was frequently dismissed and denied: You have a headache! she was told. Or, You have anxiety! Or, You have fibromyalgia! Chimére suspected it might have something to do with her identity: a Black woman in her early forties who was highly educated and had done her research. This constant dismissal became a form of structural silencing: she wasn't believed by clinicians, family members and loved ones, or society at large.

In 2022, Chimére wrote in a CNN Opinion essay, "I was used to this treatment; most doctors I spoke to since I had become ill—many of whom were White males—didn't believe I had Covid-19, preferring instead to assume I had a psychological issue. Some suspected drug use or insisted I was being abused at home."[28] After losing so much—her job, insurance, social and church groups, and—in her words—"my identity," Chimére paid a health advocate out of pocket to help her navigate the waters of the health system. Eventually it was a Black woman (resident) physician who believed her. She helped Chimére document long COVID in her medical chart and paved a path to recovery. Today Chimére has become a tour de force uniting Black long COVID survivors, and particularly women, to organize and amplify their stories in digital and policy spaces.

Recognizing embodied knowledge is even more critical when there are meaningful differences between the clinician and patient such as class, race, gender, sexuality, nationality, disability, and so on. Patient knowledge must be recognized "as knowledge" that can be embraced to contribute to better treatment.[29] Such recognition is crucial (although, sometimes harder) when a clinician may be unfamiliar with a set of symptoms, diagnoses, and existing treatments.[30] This unfamiliarity may amplify other system-level marginalization—through racism, ableism, or classism—that may cause patients harm. This is not only through incidents where patients feel unsafe or unheard; this harm is also deeply financial. Even patients like Ty are harmed when insurance companies won't reimburse clinicians who make diagnoses for unverifiable health conditions. With a limited path for recovery, insurers don't want to pay for winding journeys like Ty's. Instead, insurance companies often note that experimental treatments extend beyond the purview of medicine, dismissing possibly effective treatments as "alternative" or "nonmedical." Recognizing how such inequalities manifest in clinical contexts is imperative to improve the *experience of care* for patients, to empower clinicians to innovate around *what might work* to meet the needs of patients uniquely, and possibly to improve the *coverage for care*.

8

DISABILITY
CONSCIOUSNESS

EVERYTHING I THOUGHT I KNEW about long COVID and disability changed when my longtime mentor, colleague, and friend, Peter Brown, nearly died from Guillain-Barre syndrome, a rare neurological disorder that came on a few weeks after he had COVID-19.

In the middle of the night, Peter got up to get a glass of water. Halfway to the kitchen, his feet went out from under him. When his wife Betsy called out to him, Peter groaned, "Get me a pillow and I'll sleep here!" His body felt like Jell-O. Betsy threw him a pillow and realized something was unusually wrong. She called 911 and, although he was somewhat lucid in the ambulance, it would be several weeks until they were able to speak again.

Peter was on a ventilator in critical condition for the next month, between Thanksgiving and Christmas. We weren't sure if his diaphragm could work on its own again. Nearly forty of his past graduate students—nearly all of us anthropologists—gathered routinely to check in about his health, and with each other. It was a relief when a month later he was well enough to move from the critical intensive care unit. After a few weeks more, they removed his ventilator, and he moved to a rehabilitation facility. His diagnosis, almost immediately, was Guillain-Barre syndrome—a rare syndrome when your body's immune system attacks your nerves. Some have tingling and weakness in their hands and feet, which spreads quickly, eventually paralyzing their whole body. Peter's was the worst-case scenario. What was the trigger? SARS-CoV-2.

I had spoken with Peter several times about long COVID before he was hospitalized. This is in part because he has been my longtime mentor and colleague, so we are in constant discussion about research. Ten days before his episode, however, Peter had told me that he worried he wasn't getting better from COVID-19. "Maybe you should interview me?" Peter joked.

Peter doesn't remember anything from the weeks he was in a coma in the ICU. Although, he does remember his vivid dreams, as so many of the most serious patients do. After his diaphragm started working again, he started to breathe on his own and he slowly woke up. Peter was surrounded by his family and started to move his right side. But his left side would take much longer to recuperate. It took another four months in a rehabilitation facility to recover enough to return home, and many months thereafter to regain physical and cognitive strength. It is unimaginable to think that he could have recovered without the support of his family, especially Betsy.

My husband, Adam, and I visited Peter and Betsy over Memorial Day weekend in Atlanta. We had lunch in the cafeteria, and then Betsy gave us a tour of the Shepherd Center.[1] It was a facility founded when a wealthy family's son was immobilized after a surfing accident: there are several floors for rehabilitation, including rooms that look like typical physical therapy rooms and others that look like athletic facilities with a pool, basketball court, and gym. What struck me was when

Betsy mentioned offhand that there were so many men there, making a joke about the risk-taking motorcyclists who were rehabilitating after accidents to their spines, nerves, and brains. Some were there because of traumatic brain injuries after combat.

I smiled as we watched a group of eight thickly bearded men with tattoos covering their arms and chests doing water yoga together in Shepherd Center's pool. I saw a solitary woman sitting on a large chair being slowly lifted from the pool. As I watched her slowly ascend toward the edge of the pool, I realized how few women I'd seen around the facility despite the extraordinarily high proportion of women who are afflicted by neurological conditions; I later did some research and found that more people with spinal injuries are men.[2] Although, Peter didn't have a spinal injury; rather, his injury was to his nervous system. I could not help but wonder how sick and disabled you must be to access the facility. Moreover, I wondered *how* disability was measured and *what* types of injuries insurance would cover.

To access care and sources for recovery, you must be physically disabled enough to prove you are worthy of care and access to this extraordinary center, which is funded largely by a handful of private donors who have a personal connection to neurorehabilitation. There are only five other centers like it in the United States. If you do not have an event like Peter's, where you are fighting for your life on a ventilator, it is much harder to access the support of an arsenal of neurorehabilitation. By access, I mean not only getting a bed, but also having a clear diagnosis attached so insurance pays for it. While Peter has many advantages (he is white, male, and retired with good benefits), he also has both Medicare and supplemental insurance he received when he retired from working at a private university. In America, you cannot access good health care without a clear diagnosis and access to good insurance. Betsy told me that it is the supplemental insurance they have that financially enabled them to bring Peter to Shepherd in the first place.

The millions of people disabled by infections that have led to profound injuries to their nervous systems cannot access such a facility, in part because facilities for them do not exist, and because there is no money to support this collective healing that requires months or years of dedicated therapy. Yet, it is the amount of money that has been devoted to providing opportunities to rehabilitate from clearly visible overt neurological injuries that struck me, when so many people have been disabled by lingering invisible infections that immobilize the nervous system. When there is a slower or less visible progression toward disability, the urgency in targeted recovery does not appear to exist in the eyes of the state, medicine, or insurance companies. The slippage into sickness may be slower (or quick for some), but the lack of visibility and verifiability of their pain makes their recovery invisible too. This becomes a circular problem: limited research portfolios are dedicated to facilitating research of therapies that might aid recovery.

Feminist anthropologists Rayna Rapp and Faye Ginsburg have suggested that disability may be understood as a tension around "the drive toward an imagined and stratified biomedical utopia that fuels much recent culturally seductive medical innovation and intervention intended to fix if not cure disability."[3] In the case of Peter, there is a long road to recovery, but the interventions he can access are available to help him move toward living a healthier life. Although he will never be cured from his emotional and physical trauma, Peter continues to build strength and improve his health. In so many people's stories, however, there are very limited solutions available, in part because biomedicine translates to quick fixes like pharmaceuticals, and the gatekeepers to access facilities like Shepherd are very restricted with respect to what *type* of impairment someone experienced.

As I walked through those halls, I imagined what a rehabilitation facility for those living with a complex chronic condition like chronic Lyme, ME/CFS, or long COVID might look like. I imagined quiet rooms for meditation, steam rooms, sound therapy and massage, strength training for small subtle movements, and a warm pool for reimagining what it feels like to move freely again. This building might look like a gym, although the lights would be dimmer and quieter. There would also be a meeting room where people would share their illness odysseys to hear others' stories and convey their own.

CHRONIC LIVING IN AN INDIVIDUALIST CULTURE

Much of the care that people need is mundane. I cannot count how many times I have heard someone living with a complex chronic health condition mention how much they need someone who could help them clean their home, take a shower, take care of their cats, and cook meals that promote a healthy gut. Johanna Hedva describes these everyday costs on their philosophical blog: "When you have chronic illness, life is reduced to a relentless rationing of energy. It costs you to do anything: to get out of bed, to cook for yourself, to get dressed, to answer an email. For those without chronic illness, you can spend and spend without consequence: the cost is not a problem. For those of us with limited funds, we have to ration, we have a limited supply, we often run out before lunch."[4]

This radical transformation to everyday life brought on by a complex chronic condition requires innovation and a new "kind of living."[5] Although many people have applied for in-home help through disability and Medicaid, rarely are people who can help with these routine needs available. This requires most people to pay out of pocket for everyday tasks. This is another way in which structural silencing limits one's ability to live well with illness. When you don't have family or friends nearby who can support you, then you are left to fend for yourself.

Most people draw from the deep well of social networks and material resources they have acquired over their lifetime to remake a life amidst illness. At times, this requires that people navigate dynamics with loved ones, carers, communities, and political movements. In some cases, this is deeply reassuring and transformative. For instance, I spoke to a mom in Virginia who worked from home and had two small children. Although she had a supportive husband, her parents moved in with them for several months to care not only for her children while she was disabled, but also for her. They moved a bed to the living room because she could no longer walk up the stairs. She was an economist and rarely missed any work because she was not cognitively disabled. In fact, she told me she was so relieved she could think and write, because it fought off the depression that occasionally seeped in. However, she barely had enough energy to take a shower and walk down the stairs in the same day, let alone care for her children under five.

For others, chronic living becomes a profound trauma in itself. This trauma is situated in the unknowing and chronicity of pain, serving as an invisible mediator of well-being: you carry it with you but there is no physical weight, it activates from your subconscious when you're not expecting it, and it compounds with cumulative stress, psychological distress, and physical health in ways that you cannot understand, pushing you beyond thresholds.[6] This unknowing is amplified tenfold when you do not feel safe and cared for in your environment.

This was the case for Ruth, a white woman in her midfifties facing myriad diagnoses—ME/CFS, fibromyalgia, EBV, and long COVID—who lost her job, house, and independence when she got sick. With a limited number of options, Ruth moved two states away from her life to live with her father, a pull-yourself-up-by-your-bootstraps kind of guy. He told her she could move in but she "can't act sick around them." She told me, "I have to pretend everything is okay—it just drains the life out of you."

For Ruth, chronic living is not about living well but about surviving in a context she describes as "abusive." Every time her father tells her to get a job, anger bubbles up because her cognitive disability makes it impossible for her to work. She is counting the days until her disability goes through so she can hopefully move back on her own. However, she has already applied twice and been rejected both times. She told me that she trusted God would heal her and that she worried applying for disability was hypocritical. However, this time she got a lawyer to help her. He told her that it would be more likely she'd be granted disability if she was homeless, although she cannot imagine navigating her illness on the streets. She was very frustrated because the two reviews of her disability application were so "subjective."

I thought about Ruth when I was called for jury duty. It was a civil case—one where the plaintiff was injured while driving a county bus and was appealing a worker compensation decision that denied her coverage of medical fees. The plaintiff had worked for years as a corrections officer and had had several accidents that caused her back to ache, shoulder to stiffen, and nerves to cause tenderness. She was a low-income sixty-something Black mother residing in a rural county in Maryland and driving a bus in a bustling DC suburb. She had left the corrections department because after more than three decades, she said on the stand, she wanted "something different." It was soon clear that she'd been in several altercations with clients in her work in corrections, causing significant lower-back pain from sciatica. The county suggested that because she had pain from her previous job, the small infraction in the bus accident certainly couldn't be the root of her current suffering.

I was struck by a deposition from the plaintiff's doctor. Dr. Y spent 45 minutes explaining the biology of sciatic pain, deciphering movement and duress according to an MRI. Near the end of an exhausting cross-examination, where the prosecutor homed in on minor differences between two MRIs spaced a decade apart, Dr. Y's eyes lingered on the papers on his desk. He looked up at the lawyer and stated something like, "Well, pain is subjective. Even if we don't see something on the MRI, a patient can be in pain that is debilitating." I could barely contain my shock when this doctor concluded, after hours of trying to prove something visible and measurable determined the plaintiff's pain, that we in fact may never know how much pain she was in.

The jury voted in favor of the plaintiff. In deliberation, I suggested, "Why don't we just believe her?" Many others agreed—that her pain was preexisting but the accident, as minor as it was, exacerbated her suffering. This was after a certain amount of deliberation about what it means to believe people's pain in the first place. I wonder what the conversation might have been like if I had not spent the last year writing this book, spending hour upon hour listening to people's stories about the depth of pain in their heads, necks, backs, muscles, stomachs, tissues, and elsewhere that stayed with them. None of this pain was *visible* to others. How many plaintiffs are dismissed because it's unclear that an accident was "severe" enough to cause pain that is verifiable?

VISIBLE GRIEF

I have often discussed the chronicity of physical pain, but living through a radical health transition can also carry with it deep emotional pain, particularly when the political environment is as chaotic and uncertain as your health. A woman I call Sam, who is Black and in her midtwenties, got sick in the earliest days of the pandemic when she was working in a nursing home in Atlanta. She recalled, "Everyone was dying all around us." Many of her patients got sick and went to the hospital. Most didn't come back, and those who did were on oxygen and barely living. The emotional trauma of that work was stark: people were getting sick and being removed regularly, leaving the nursing staff heartsick and exhausted.[7]

Sam was infected with COVID-19 first in April and then again in May of 2020. The second time was so intense, Sam's mother, living in Illinois, called Atlanta 911 for her. Sam described the relief she felt from the oxygen during the ambulance ride. By the time she got to the hospital, she was barely conscious. She went into a coma and was hospitalized for thirty-six days.

Sam's near-death experience has changed the way she sees herself, and the world. She had fever dreams and an intense spiritual experience of living and dying, staying and going, being and moving on. She explained, "One of the first things I remember was this voice—I don't know what she said, but I understood it was my body—do you want to stay, or do you want to go? I was confused—stay or go, and the next thing I remember I was on stage, and I was singing . . . 'All That Jazz.' . . . I couldn't see my family, but I remember hearing them. I was telling them, I'm right here." She felt she was outside of her body, looking down and deciding whether to leave her corporeal life. She said: "I was talking to the virus, and it was telling me, I just want to survive. And I was just like, yeah, you should live. And my ancestors told me, what are you doing here? You shouldn't be here."

George Floyd's murder, a violent injustice against a Black man that catalyzed a major social movement organized online and in the streets, happened during Sam's hospitalization. She doesn't know whether it was because of the hospital televisions constantly blaring news in the background, or because of her near-death experience, but she feels deeply connected to that moment in time. Floyd's murder was emotionally and politically significant to her as a Black woman living in the United States, but she also had a spiritual connection to his death because she felt that she, too, had died when his body left this earth. She remembers saying, "Stay here, we matter. We deserve to be here."

Sam recalls people praying for her while she was comatose. However, she doesn't know if people were praying for her in her hospital room, or if her ancestors prayed for her spiritual body, or if any prayers protected her at all. Regardless, her memories have become a central part of how she makes sense of a time of extraordinary fracture.

Understanding the structural and societal realities of this moment in time is crucial to making sense of Sam's experience. The depth of her trauma and chronic pain is not linked to her genetic predisposition, but linked to the multifactored ways in which COVID-19 uniquely impacted

Black Americans. Essential workers carried a disproportionate exposure risk in the early pandemic, and Black Americans held a disproportionate number of essential worker positions.[8] In the United States, one-third of licensed practical and vocational nurses are Black, meaning a disproportionate number of Black people had early exposure to not only the virus, but early pandemic trauma.[9] Black Americans also died at higher rates and suffered greater psychological trauma from personal exposures and grief.[10]

However, not all pain and grief are medically related. When Sam was released from the hospital, her parents drove down to Atlanta to bring her home to Illinois so they could care for her. Sam described the shame and regret she carried with her about leaving her adopted city. She earned her LPN and was working in a job she loved in a new city she'd discovered and enjoyed. She had built a community, had her own apartment, and created a life for herself. After she got sick, she couldn't live on her own anymore—at least not for now, they thought. They left her stuff in her Atlanta apartment and continued paying the rent for several months until they realized there was no way she could return to the life she once lived there. After sinking thousands of dollars into rent, her family got a U-Haul and moved her things to her parents' house.

Sam felt a lot of anger for a long time following her hospitalization. Part of this anger was linked to her trouble breathing—every day she would relive her trauma. Whenever she struggled to breathe normally, she was reminded of what happened to her. In her mind, Sam wove together the injustice of her hospitalization with the injustice of George Floyd's murder and the uprisings that happened throughout the summer of 2020. She says that her anger was triggered by something "small," and she realized that she couldn't live in this world this way. She needed to deal with her anger so she could find calm in the wake of the storm.

Once she was settled in Illinois, Sam started physical therapy and lung therapy. She had a good primary care doctor but struggled to establish specialty care for her breathing. At first, her pulmonologist said her problems were related to her weight, meaning her respiratory problems were a consequence of being "fat." This type of discriminatory fatphobia is common in medicine, where some symptoms are attributed to weight as opposed to other treatable health conditions.[11] After the pulmonologist ordered X-rays and a lung function test, he apologized and said that her symptoms were real, and her lungs were in bad shape. In some ways, he realized that he had brought discriminatory bias to the examination room and doing so had deeply affected his patient. Sam is confident and advocated for herself—over time they have built trust, and he has become an important clinician supporting her recovery.

Four years later, Sam continues to need routine rehabilitation and care. For several months, she would seek care at the clinic, but now she only sees her primary care doctor every four to six months. Early in her recovery, Sam would fall frequently—her legs buckling beneath her, causing great alarm to herself and her family. Moving helped her manage muscle pain, but it was awful and consistent. This muscular pain is one of the most pervasive and consistent symptoms that she's carried since her infection—apart from the emotional trauma. Her physical therapy insurance coverage ended after only a few sessions; thankfully, her parents were able to pay out of pocket for her physical therapy for several months through a hospital program so that Sam could build the strength she needed to reimagine her life. Coupled with online group counseling, Sam found meaningful work and a newfound joy that is radically unlike what she expected for her life before she got sick. With her family's help, Sam has been able to cultivate a new normal.

FINDING A NEW PACE

How people push on while living with complex chronic illness is a crucial element in thinking about recovery, in part because life after infection may look very different than before. As I have argued throughout the book, recovery with a complex chronic illness is not about a *cure* because there is none, although some people go into remission. Rather, it's about reestablishing a new baseline and pace in life—about reimagining what a good life means while managing the waves of illness.

In 2023, Jim Jackson published a book, *Clearing the Fog*, which was based on his work with a long COVID community from some of the earliest stages.[12] Before the world shut down, Jackson, who is a psychologist, was working with people suffering from post-intensive care syndrome (PICS), a condition where health problems that may involve physical pain, thoughts, feelings, or cognition remain after critical illness. These lingering effects of critical illness affect not only the patient, but also the family. Jackson quickly adapted his therapeutic practice for long COVID patients. "It was sort of like that homage, if you build it, they will come," he said. I spoke to several people in Jackson's support groups. These groups literally saved people's lives. "I thought a lot of other places would embrace this kind of psychology-led support group model," he told me. "I felt sure that it would really proliferate. That really hasn't happened. So that's been a little bit of a disappointment, I think, because our program has worked so well. We have an interdisciplinary team."

I met many people like Sam through Jackson's team after I reached out to them about recruiting patients with varied experiences and backgrounds. At the time, his new book was making the rounds and everyone was texting me, "Did you see this NPR interview with Jim Jackson?" Ruth explained how these support groups were the one place she felt believed and encouraged to find joy. She explained, "Dr. Jackson's very compassionate and knows what we are going through. Most people don't believe us and don't understand what we're going through. But Dr. Jackson has something special about him and he gets it. And getting on the calls with other people who are experiencing the same thing can be helpful. It can also be depressing—when I see others in the groups struggling even more than I am. . . . Dr. Jackson talks about acceptance—this is where I am today, and I think I might do one little thing that can bring some joy."

The long COVID recovery journey differs in such meaningful ways among people. "What I generally find is that it's not a straight line of improvement," an infectious disease physician and researcher told me. This researcher started following long COVID patients in 2020, when people she'd long followed in her clinic started presenting with symptoms. She explained, "It's a jagged trend of relapses. The general trend is that people are getting better." However, most people don't bounce back to the same health state they had before they were sick. A long-time policy expert working in health for the government—turned long-hauler—described to me how people living with long COVID are adapting to living with the condition rather than returning to their baseline before infection. He described how one colleague, for example, paced her way back to work—coming back part- and then full-time. But to do this, she would spend every Saturday in bed. And even though it looks like she's resumed her work life, that life is very different from the one she led before she got sick.

I spoke to a nurse I call Nell in Canada who worked through five COVID-19 infections and felt her health slipping away. She was on the brink of despair. One of her five adult children stopped by one day and encouraged her to engage in radical rest. "I had to dial back on everything in my life to find a cocktail that worked for me," Nell told me. "I stopped everything—I gave myself permission to feel sick. To not pressure myself to feel better. I gave myself permission to take days off and focus on myself. It's hard to do that because you feel like you're letting everyone down in your life. If you're not good to yourself, you can't be good for anyone else. I needed to get better, and I knew what I needed to do." At one point, Nell bought a ticket to a small beach resort in Mexico and spent two weeks engaged in radical rest, basking in the sun, eating fresh fruits, and doing nothing more than letting her body heal. While planning this trip brought her spirits up, she realized that positive thinking and meditation were making her feel stronger.

Nell doesn't consider herself a long-hauler, in part because her illness experience has radically changed. "I cut out all caffeine, supplements, and went to the basics of what I needed, like my iron gets low. I tried to push as much water and close-to-the-ground type of eating as possible. I'd go on walks. I did a liver cleanse twice. I felt a boost of energy and felt like the clouds parted for me. I felt clean energy—on the inside. After doing the detox, I feel more energized and I feel like everything has been flushed out of my system. I just eat fruits and vegetables—I took out red meat. I eat fish and chicken. I set up a routine and have a set bedtime. Oh, my, I cannot tell you how many days of work I missed."

In part because of this winding road, many people with complex chronic conditions have opted out of conventional medical care in search of their own remedies that address syndromic conditions and enable them to reimagine a full life. This looks very different for everyone.

Bethany's experience improved once she was able to secure disability, save her house, and secure in-house help to keep her environment clean and calm. Once Lena received her long COVID diagnosis, she felt more settled understanding what could be triggering her dysregulation and how to manage her symptoms. Molly unfortunately is consumed with managing a new health crisis, surrounded by the support and love of her family. Tam stays optimistic and manages her health carefully, taking a rainbow of pills every day and monitoring her environment and stress load. Ken has largely recovered and received a prestigious scholarship for medical school; he still experiences fatigue and migraines from time to time. Jo is writing fiercely to elevate the experience of trans people living with disabilities. JD is now in a master's program focused on writing so he can more strategically tell his own story of patient activism. Chimére is filming her documentary on Black women's experiences living with long COVID in America. Ty is managing his cancer diagnosis with the support of his family. Ja'Mia is handling her health day by day, as she has since she was young. Sam is doing well and found a new job that pays okay; she engages with people (from a safe distance) and continues to rely on the online therapy groups Jackson and others offer. Peter is back to his old self, although his mobility doesn't look the same as before he got sick. I grin ear to ear every time I see a text from him.

CONCLUSION

IN JANUARY OF 1892, American writer Charlotte Perkins Stetson published a semi-autobiographical short story, "The Yellow Wall-Paper," which captured an experience of neurasthenia.[1] In the story, she was prescribed the rest cure,
requiring women to lay down their pens, paintbrushes, and
books to overcome their nervous weakness. In the essay,
Stetson described how the cure itself drove one to melancholia, excising any form of power they might have had
before their sickness drove them to prescribed isolation. Her
writing about the humiliating experience of this treatment
in *New England Magazine* had a profound impact on how people perceived neurasthenia and how clinicians treated it.
Some clinicians admitted later that they would never pre-
scribe the rest cure again, noting how debilitating the isolation alone can be.

More than a century later, we are telling the same stories
with different medical idioms and social situations. A major

difference now is that, in many cases, we have a deeper understanding of the possible variations of health conditions that share similar symptoms and illness trajectories. Multiple sclerosis is not categorized as hysteria, for example, because we can see plaque built up in the brain. But those conditions that still lack verifiability remain in a liminal state of legitimacy—something that is perpetuated because we do not have the scientific expertise to understand how viruses persist and dysregulate, or how to mitigate their effects.

Yet, we have patient expertise. I found Johanna Hedva's account of "Sick Woman Theory," which I refer to throughout the book, to be one of the most philosophically and experientially cogent frames of what it is like to live with these health conditions, not only in the corporeal body, but also in society, politics, and medicine. Using this knowledge and experience as research—despite the small number of data points—could be a powerful conduit to generate a deeper understanding of patient needs. In other words, how do we elevate the in-depth experiences of complex patients to be recognized as legitimate sources of knowledge?

Long COVID has opened a window for a health care revolution, although much more needs to be done. Shifting *what* type of expertise matters, *who* is viewed as legitimately sick, and *how* people can receive the care they desperately need is an urgent concern that has for too long been kicked to the back of the list of priorities in medicine. Part of the problem is that the medical model that doggedly and narrowly envisions *cure* and *recovery* may overlook or obscure the wisdom of people's bodies. We need more solutions that are bold and creative, thinking outside the box and revisiting what is possible to calm the body and help people find a new and functional normal. Building on the decades of research of patient-activists and scholars who have devoted their lives—often from the confines of their beds—to generating knowledge and understanding that can help themselves and others is the starting point medicine needs to radically transform how patients are received, cared for, and imagined in clinical contexts.

REIMAGINING CARE

There are several examples of what we *could* do with the political and financial support of the people. Without a doubt, this would require a government who cares deeply about providing equitable health care and recognizes the value of human life. Disability activist, anthropologist, and theologian Erin Raffety described four critical ways to elevate ease and access for people living with dynamic disabilities. I found these four strategies to be very useful to think with, particularly considering what is possible in the current political and social system that for so long has elevated profits over people and focused on specialization over complexity.

First, it's crucial to adapt the environment so that the social and structural spaces people navigate are safe and accessible for all. It's not only ramps, elevators, and braille directives that make an environment accessible, but also a slew of other technologies, from digital to emotional, which can make an environment more accessible. This might include a dark and quiet space to rest during a meeting, a sensory room for people to calm their nervous systems, and reliable virtual meeting options for people who are not well enough to attend in person.

Second, adapt the process people must go through to access accommodations in the first place. The extensive bureaucratic hoops many people must jump through to access accommodations can be extraordinary and uneven: so many people I spoke to described how their disability coverage was only approved after hiring a lawyer to manage the labyrinth of paperwork. This is particularly difficult when you are living with dynamic disability, where you are too sick to work but may look well. While these accommodations include Social Security Disability Insurance, they also include health coverage options such as Medicaid and Medicare. No patient living with a chronic illness should be left unhoused, hungry, afraid, and alone due to illness. Although, we know that today thousands of long COVID patients have lost their jobs, homes, and health, and the safety net is failing them.

Third, increase accessibility to products and tools people need to navigate the world, from wheelchairs to hearing aids and digital tools. These tools need to be affordable and accessible for everyone to use them; adapting to a new life where a wheelchair or other mobility devices might enhance the quality of life can be a game changer, even if someone is physically mobile but exhausts easily. On the other hand, ensuring that people have access to digital tools (like phones) where they can access a video, the internet, and a phone to speak to their doctor, work, or social circles, especially on days when they are resting, is fundamental for living well with dynamic disability.

Finally, providing comprehensive medical care is essential. This final accommodation made me think about how flipping the medical model on its head is crucial to provide good care for people living with complex chronic conditions. I found Alba Azola's description of what this looks like in practice to be most useful to think with. Azola is a physiatrist at Johns Hopkins University who spends most of her time today serving patients in the Chronic Fatigue Syndrome Clinic at JHU Hospital that was originally founded by a pioneer in the field, Peter Rowe. However, for years she worked with patients rehabilitating from surgery, traumatic brain injury, critical illness, spinal cord injury, and strokes. During the pandemic they launched a Post-COVID Clinic, first working with critically ill patients in the ICU and then shifting to outpatient care for people living with long COVID. Azola found extraordinary meaning in this work and has worked with long COVID patients ever since.

Azola detailed what clinics for people living with complex chronic conditions must look like to facilitate better care for patients on their own terms. This means that issues like safe housing, transportation, access to healthy foods, and social support must be considered insurable treatments. This level of insurance is both fundamental for accessing care and possibly the largest hurdle because insurance drives everything in American medicine. Clinicians must be able to identify what resources patients have at their disposal, from medical or scientific training to patient advocacy groups and access to other types of healers. Such understanding is particularly delicate when caring for people who may face more discrimination than others, particularly women, children, trans people, people living with a disability, and the uninsured. In many ways this involves centering patient knowledge, experience, and positionality—something that is largely uncomfortable when clinicians are trained in a system that encourages them to perceive themselves, above all, as experts. However, in this case, respectful dialogue is foundational, particularly when patient expertise in rarer conditions is crucial to identify the multi-systems problems and solutions.

One way to support patients is through better training for medical students and practitioners around complex chronic conditions. #MEAction's new campaign called #TeachMETreatME, for example, focuses on elevating medical education for clinicians generally. A broader education about complex chronic conditions—addressing issues of complexity specifically—is fundamental for changing clinicians' ability to identify, diagnose, and treat patients with such conditions. Lack of knowledge can shape and bias future clinical encounters by writing misrepresentations into charts and referrals that shape symptom interpretations, including erroneous diagnoses. For instance, writing "functional neurological disorder" in a patient's medical chart may set the course for future treatment, causing clinicians to wonder if a patient is telling the truth about their symptoms in every future clinical encounter. A diagnosis of FND can set back patient care for months, if not years, particularly when their condition is associated with a virus or bacterial infection. This is complicated more by the lack of a verifiable test or sign for diagnosis.

It might be that even a new residency program is required for physicians interested in tackling this extraordinary challenge of complex chronic conditions. The residency program would be situated within the ideals of precision medicine, where treatment prescriptions are formulated around unique needs of patients. However, what is considered to be treatment would expand beyond the common frame of "genetics, environment, and lifestyle" to include more holistic thought about patient backgrounds, environments, life experiences, collections of symptoms and triggers, routines, social networks, and financial needs. This program would be organized around the principle that illness experiences are fundamentally framed by a patient's unique Venn diagram of symptoms and diagnoses. Specifically, orienting some training around the concept of "septad" conditions—the notion that complex chronic health conditions are often made up of multiple diagnoses that are cross-linked—will facilitate fundamental understanding of people's illness and healing needs.[2] Training a cadre of clinicians focusing on this complexity would be a radical shift in modern medicine and provide an opportunity for social transformation in how such health conditions are perceived and treated in the medical field.

Clinical contexts for people living with complex chronic conditions must coordinate interdisciplinary teams that have space to discuss their cases generously at length and over time. The optimal clinical context, Azola described to me, involves knowledgeable providers, including specialists, who can move in and out of a clinical room during an elongated session with a patient. This might also include clinics where holistic and integrative practitioners can work across biological and health systems. It might require practitioners who are trained to implement holistic approaches for evaluating patients and coordinating multidisciplinary care for people (as opposed to conventional medical subspecialists who are so narrowly focused on one part of the body). In this scenario, patients would be able to travel to the clinic or hospital fewer times, which would ultimately improve their health and save everyone money. It would also require a team or collaborative care approach focused on the unique social, psychological, and physical needs of the patient. Some patients, especially those dealing with mobility issues, may benefit from the return to house visits so that they can save their energy for healing.

This scenario might also employ patient consultants who are knowledgeable about unverifiable health conditions to serve as knowledge partners. Clinical researchers often note the importance of recognizing and possibly understanding the lived experiences of patients. However, many people do not believe this approach is enough to transform the practice of medicine to be more inclusive and effective in caring for people. Rather, it's crucial that people living with invisible illness are recognized and integrated into clinical and research teams as knowledge partners. Patients offer invaluable knowledge, from experiential to scientific, that should be viewed with as much "openness and rigor as other forms of knowledge."[3]

This returns us to the vital question: what is health? As we move farther from the pandemic period, and possibly toward the next one, rethinking dichotomies of deservingness is imperative: *good* health and *ill*-health, abled and dis-abled, strong and weak, wealthy and impoverished. Making sense of how people remake a life in a bodymind that is forever changed can be an extraordinary challenge. Finding a new balance and understanding of what health is amidst illness is one way many people cultivate a sense of self. Yet, remaking a life with illness involves much more than the self—it requires a community who believes them: a friend to call them back, bills to be paid, bellies to be filled, a secure home to live in, reliable and affordable psychotherapy and rehabilitation support, and a health system they can rely on.

Acknowledgments

EVERYTHING WE WRITE BUILDS on the experience, knowledge, and intuition of those who came before us and walk beside us. I am grateful to everyone who shared spoons to feed my knowledge to write this book and convey their stories. I am especially grateful to those people who spoke to me in their moments of feeling well and with clarity—as I know in some cases those moments are rare. I am also indebted to colleagues who shared their life stories alongside their research, providing nuance to the complex ways in which people uncover truth and how essential such experts are as knowledge partners.

To write this book, I needed a moment to breathe. I am indebted to the John Simon Guggenheim Memorial Foundation for believing in this project and selecting me to take a break and focus my energy on it. I was exhausted and overstretched from raising two young children and working as a medical anthropologist investigating COVID-19 during the early pandemic years. The Guggenheim Fellowship gave me the space I needed to practice yoga, get lost in my community pottery studio, care for my children in deep and rejuvenating ways, and write this book. Having a sabbatical is a rare gift, and I savored every minute of it.

I spent a wonderful afternoon discussing an earlier draft of this work with a critical collective of scholars and activists working on complex chronic illnesses. This workshop was hosted by the Medical Humanities program at Georgetown University, and I thank my lucky stars for the kindness, support, and laughs I've shared over the years with my friends Timothy Newfield and Lakshmi Krishnan. I was so grateful to Rayna Rapp, Emily Lim Rogers, and Jaime Seltzer for traveling to DC for the workshop. Rayna gave incredibly deep and reflective insights, gently suggesting I read deeper and more broadly on disability. Many comments Emily provided—both practical and theoretical—are sprinkled throughout the book and I am grateful to have engaged with them. Also, Jaime's sharp reading and deep understanding of the patient activism community were essential. Thank you to my DC collective of scholars and friends who joined in the discussion, most (but not all) of whom are at Georgetown. Thank you to Dhruvi Banerjee, Lydia X. Z. Brown, Caroline Efird, Bruce Gellin, Amy Kenny, Jake Lang, Sylvia Önder, Cora Salkovskis, Rachel Singer, and Emilia Guevara for engaging with the work so deeply and providing such constructive and critical feedback. Separately, I am appreciative to Arthur Kleinman for engaging deeply in this manuscript with me and encouraging me to rewrite a few sections. A final point of gratitude is for Libbie Rifkin who provided key feedback at the right moment.

As I was making last-minute edits, I decided to pilot the book with my students enrolled in my course Mind, Madness, Meditation. I never imagined how fun it would be. They jumped in with two feet, providing immensely insightful comments and help with some last-minute organization of ideas. It was a delightful two hours of workshopping this book. Thank you to Dhruvi Banerjee, Cassie Clark, Bailey Coghlan, Kayla Dunn, Esha Gupta, Cassius Hou, Nina Jennings, Jake Lang, Liya Lin, Camila Navarro-Delavega, Lili Rodgers, Freddy Rodriguez, Abbey Schiller, Saatvik Sunkavalli, and Marie Tetsu. After we discussed the book, we all lay on the floor together for a 25-minute meditation and I'm certain, at least at that point, that I heard some soft snoring.

Everything falls into place when you find the right editor. I'm grateful for what Elise Capron did to move this book forward, and for the thoughtful editing and encouragement from Kate Marshall and her team at University of California Press. The anonymous reviewers she recruited also provided gentle probing to rework sections of the book. This was essential and at the right time.

I have a very strong support network of readers in my community. I am so thankful for their encouragement for writing this book and reminders of what a broad audience might want to know. A special thanks to aunt, mom, and cousins (Abby Adams, Barb Mendenhall, John Bowers, and Isabelle Gigante) who pushed me to think about all sides. A special thanks to my friend Mike Ebinger, who reminded me how important this work is for people close to me.

Partners of any kind—spouses, canines, colleagues—play a special role in writing. My partner Adam has an unusual amount of patience and balance, and I'm grateful to him, our girls Fiona and Zoë, and our pups, for bringing equal amounts of chaos and dynamism, love and joy, and particularly good distraction to my life. I love you all so much.

Notes

A GLOSSARY OF CONDITIONS

1. Price, "The Bodymind Problem and the Possibilities of Pain."
2. Liptan, "Fascia."
3. *Septad* was coined by Ilene Ruhoy, a neurologist at Mount Sinai South in New York. https://spinalcsfleak.org/dr-ilene-ruhoy-complex-patient/.

INTRODUCTION

1. Reynolds, "They Never Officially Had COVID-19. Months Later They're Living in Hell."
2. Hedva, "Sick Woman Theory."
3. Mingus, "Access Intimacy: The Missing Link."
4. Davis et al., "Long COVID."
5. Price, "The Bodymind Problem and the Possibilities of Pain," 269.
6. Latour, *Reassembling the Social.*

7. Lock, "Comprehending the Body in the Era of the Epigenome," 156.

8. Davis et al., "Long COVID."

9. Sapolsky, *Why Zebras Don't Get Ulcers*; Mendenhall, *Rethinking Diabetes*.

10. Geronimus, "The Weathering Hypothesis and the Health of African American Women and Infants"; Geronimus, "Black/White Differences in the Relationship of Maternal Age to Birthweight."

11. McEwen, "Stress, Adaptation, and Disease."

12. Sharma and Bayry, "High Risk of Autoimmune Diseases after COVID-19."

13. This common term in medical anthropology—*diagnostic odyssey*—was coined by Frank in *The Wounded Storyteller*.

14. Dumes, *Divided Bodies*.

15. Barnes, *The Minority Body*; Barnes, *Health Problems*.

16. Mendenhall, *Unmasked*.

17. Patient activist Amy Watson coined the term "long-hauler" in April 2020 to reference patients whose symptoms persisted for weeks and months. She was wearing a hat when she got tested, after she wasn't recovering, that said "Long Haul." Soon after, she started one of the first Facebook groups for people with persistent conditions, which grew quickly.

18. Brown et al., "Embodied Health Movements."

19. Epstein, *Impure Science*, 8.

20. Prior, *The Long Haul*.

21. Wahlberg, "Serious Disease as Kinds of Living"; Manderson and Wahlberg, "Chronic Living in a Communicable World"; Manderson et al., *Viral Loads*.

22. Wendell, "Unhealthy Disabled."

23. Zabiliūtė and McNeilly, "Relational Chronicities."

24. Ware, "Suffering and the Social Construction of Illness"; Ware, "Toward a Model of Social Course in Chronic Illness."

25. Refer to the following for a more extensive discussion of signs and symptoms in unverifiable chronic illnesses: Dumes, *Divided Bodies*.

26. Dumes, *Divided Bodies*.

27. Packard et al., *Emerging Illnesses and Society*; Dumes, *Divided Bodies*.

28. Kirmayer, "Beyond the 'New Cross-cultural Psychiatry'"; Keller, *Refiguring Life.*

29. Hsu et al., "Patients as Knowledge Partners in the Context of Complex Chronic Conditions."

30. Dysautonomia can feature in a number of health conditions, from Parkinson's disease and Ehlers-Danlos syndrome (EDS) to HIV/AIDS, autism, postural orthostatic tachycardia syndrome (POTS), ME/CFS, and long COVID.

31. These frictions emerged within and between interviews with patients and clinicians. Discussions with two clinicians living with complex chronic illness made this clearer. Leah Ratner works with pediatric patients living with verifiable illnesses like cerebral palsy and explains that many things are similar with her patients, but there are significant differences when something is unverifiable. Zeest Khan, an anesthesiologist who was disabled by long COVID, has become a long COVID educator and activist. She explained that in her experience, patients and clinicians are speaking across each other.

32. Lock and Nguyen, *An Anthropology of Biomedicine.*

33. We have published some of this work we did together: Kaplan and Mendenhall, "Framing Long Covid through Patient Activism in the United States"; Mendenhall and Kaplan, "The 'Brain Fog' of Long COVID Is a Serious Medical Issue That Needs More Attention."

34. Among the patients, one-third were low-income, one-third were middle-income, and one-third were upper-middle- or high-income. Two-thirds were white; the rest self-identified as Black, Indian, Indigenous, Iranian, Latinx, or Taiwanese. Of the seventy-one people who identified as patients among the people I interviewed, two-thirds were white and one-third were not, including mostly Black and Latinx voices. Of the people interviewed, 80 percent identified as women, 13 percent as male, and 4 percent as nonbinary or trans. Because of the imbalance in my sample, I read closely reports put together by patient advocacy groups representing nonwhite voices, to garner a broader and deeper understanding of patient perspectives.

35. Crenshaw, "Demarginalizing the Intersection of Race and Sex," 139. Intersectionality is a bedrock of intellectual framing for many Black feminist health scholars such as Whitney Pirtle, Hanna Garth, and Ashanté Reese; one

good resource is to look through the Cite Black Women collective, https:// www.citeblackwomencollective.org/our-collective.html.

CHAPTER ONE

1. Wilson, *Psychosomatic.*

2. Kleinman, *Social Origins of Distress and Disease,* 59.

3. Griffith, *The Petrie Papyri.*

4. Edwards, "Hysteria."

5. Tasca et al., "Women and Hysteria in the History of Mental Health."

6. Shorter, *From Paralysis to Fatigue,* 17.

7. Cleghorn, *Unwell Women,* 64.

8. Cleghorn, *Unwell Women,* 64.

9. Cleghorn, *Unwell Women,* 63.

10. Cleghorn, *Unwell Women,* 64–65.

11. Shorter, *From Paralysis to Fatigue,* 5.

12. Shorter, *From Paralysis to Fatigue,* 12.

13. Shorter, *From Paralysis to Fatigue,* 21.

14. Shorter, *From Paralysis to Fatigue,* 22.

15. Cleghorn, *Unwell Women,* 99.

16. Tilt, *On Diseases of Menstruation and Ovarian Inflammation.* In Cleghorn, *Unwell Women,* 101–2.

17. Cleghorn, *Unwell Women,* 101–2.

18. Brigo, "Jean-Martin Charcot (1825–1893) and His Second Thoughts about Hysteria."

19. Wilson, *Psychosomatic.*

20. Charcot, *Leçons du Mardi à la Salpêtrière (1887–1888),* quoted in Shorter, *From Paralysis to Fatigue.*

21. Lerner, *Hysterical Men.*

22. Wilson, *Psychosomatic.*

23. Breuer and Freud, *Studies on Hysteria.*

24. Wilson, *Psychosomatic,* 31.

25. Webster, "Freud, Charcot, and Hysteria."

26. Lunden, *American Breakdown.*

27. Maybin et al., "COVID-19 and Abnormal Uterine Bleeding."

28. Davis, *Reproductive Injustice.*

29. Beard, "Neurasthenia, or Nervous Exhaustion."

30. Beard, *American Nervousness.*

31. Beard, *A Practical Treatise on Nervous Exhaustion (Neurasthenia).*

32. Schuster, *Neurasthenic Nation,* 27–30.

33. Allbutt, "Nervous Diseases and Modern Life"; quoted in Greenwood, "Looking Back."

34. Schuster, *Neurasthenic Nation,* 3.

35. Beard, *American Nervousness,* 13, 56.

36. Schuster, *Neurasthenic Nation,* 27.

37. Wessely, "Old Wine in New Bottles."

38. Marcus, "ONE STEP BACK: Where Are the Elixirs of Yesteryear When We Hurt?"

39. Musser and Kelly, *A Handbook of Practical Treatment.*

40. Schuster, *Neurasthenic Nation.*

41. Goetz, "Poor Beard!!"

42. Cleghorn, *Unwell Women,* 116.

43. Van Deusen, "Observations on a Form of Nervous Prostration."

44. Mitchel, *Wear and Tear,* 33, quoted in Cleghorn, *Unwell Women,* 116.

45. Kirmayer, "Mind and Body as Metaphors," 57.

46. Scheper-Hughes and Lock, "The Mindful Body."

47. Cleghorn, *Unwell Women,* 101.

48. Chambers, "Clinical Lecture on Hysteria," in Cleghorn, *Unwell Women,* 102.

49. Chrichton Miller, *Functional Nerve Disease.*

50. Shorter, *From Paralysis to Fatigue,* 221.

51. Taylor, "A Study of Neurasthenia at the National Hospital for the Relief and Cure of the Paralysed and Epileptic."

52. Putnam Jacobi, *Essays on Hysteria,* 63–64, quoted in Shorter, *From Paralysis to Fatigue,* 223–24.

53. Cleghorn, *Unwell Women,* 133–35.

54. Putnam Jacobi, *The Question of Rest for Women during Menstruation;* Cleghorn, *Unwell Women,* 113–15.

55. Wilson, *Psychosomatic,* 97.

56. Showalter, *Hystories.*

57. Showalter, *Hystories.*

58. Wilson, *Psychosomatic*, 13.

59. Spinney, *Pale Rider*, 13–14.

60. Spinney, *Pale Rider*, 14.

61. Spinney, *Pale Rider*, 19–21.

62. Krishnan, "An Extraordinary Sequel," 303.

63. Krishnan, "An Extraordinary Sequel," 303.

64. Putnam Jacobi, "Hysterical Fever."

65. Krishnan, "An Extraordinary Sequel," 305.

66. Krishnan, "An Extraordinary Sequel," 307.

67. Krishnan, "An Extraordinary Sequel," 307.

68. Honigsbaum and Krishnan, "Taking Pandemic Sequelae Seriously."

69. Barry, *The Great Influenza.*

70. Phillips and Killingray, *The Spanish Influenza Pandemic of 1918–1919*, 11–13.

71. See Ravenhold, "Encephalitis Lethargica," 708–13.

72. Phillips, *In a Time of Plague.*

73. Patterson and Pyle, "The Diffusion of Influenza in Sub-Saharan Africa during the 1918–1919 Pandemic."

74. Phillips, *Black October.*

75. Ellison, "A Fierce Hunger," 225.

76. Ellison, "A Fierce Hunger," 224, 293.

77. Gilliam, *Epidemiological Study of an Epidemic.*

78. Bruno et al., "Parallels between Post-Polio Fatigue and Chronic Fatigue Syndrome."

79. Sharif et al., "On Chronic Fatigue Syndrome and Nosological Categories."

80. Rosenow et al., "Observations on the Epidemic of Polio-Encephalitis in Los Angeles."

81. Sigurdsson, Fridbjorn, "History of ME and Long Covid," presentation of personally shared slides following a discussion at the National Institutes of Health meeting on what long COVID can learn from ME/CFS, June 2023.

82. Marinacci and Von Hagen, "The Value of the Electromyogram in the Diagnosis of Iceland Disease."

83. Blattner, "Benign Myalgic Encephalomyelitis (Akureyri Disease, Iceland Disease)."

84. Sharif et al., "On Chronic Fatigue Syndrome and Nosological Categories."

85. Sigurdsson and Gudmundsson, "Clinical Findings Six Years after Outbreak of Akureyri Disease"; Parish, "Early Outbreaks of 'Epidemic Neuromyasthenia.'"

86. Líndal et al., "Anxiety Disorders."

87. Pellew, "A Clinical Description of a Disease Resembling Poliomyelitis."

88. Hyde and Bergmann, "Akureyri Disease (Myalgic Encephalomyelitis), Forty Years Later."

89. Ramsay, "'Epidemic Neuromyasthenia' 1955–1978."

90. Lancet, "A New Clinical Entity?"

91. Ramsay, "Hysteria and 'Royal Free Disease.'"

92. McEvedy and Beard, "Royal Free Epidemic of 1955."

93. Committee on the Diagnostic Criteria for Myalgic Encephalomyelitis/Chronic Fatigue Syndrome, *Beyond Myalgic Encephalomyelitis/Chronic Fatigue Syndrome*; Underhill and Baillod, "Myalgic Encephalomyelitis/Chronic Fatigue Syndrome."

94. Ramsay, *Myalgic Encephalomyelitis and Postviral Fatigue States.*

CHAPTER TWO

1. "160 Victims at Lake Tahoe."

2. Johnson, *Osler's Web*. These characterizations are also included in the #MEPedia entry entitled, "1984 Incline Village Chronic Fatigue Syndrome Outbreak." https://me-pedia.org/wiki/1984_Incline_Village_chronic_fatigue_syndrome_outbreak.

3. Johnson, *Osler's Web.*

4. Johnson, *Osler's Web*, 53.

5. Johnson reports ten patients; however, a relevant *JAMA* article reports fifteen: Holmes et al., "A Cluster of Patients with a Chronic Mononucleosis-Like Syndrome."

6. Aronowitz, "From Myalgic Encephalitic to Yuppie Flu," 161–64.

7. Holmes et al., "Chronic Fatigue Syndrome: A Working Case Definition."

8. Committee on the Diagnostic Criteria for Myalgic Encephalomyelitis/Chronic Fatigue Syndrome, *Beyond Myalgic Encephalomyelitis.*

9. Holmes et al., "A Cluster of Patients with a Chronic Mononucleosis-Like Syndrome."

10. Holmes et al., "Chronic Fatigue Syndrome."

11. FDA, *The Voice of the Patient.*

12. Jason et al., "Stigma and the Term Chronic Fatigue Syndrome"; Jason and Richman, "How Science Can Stigmatize."

13. Jason and Richman, "How Science Can Stigmatize."

14. Johnson, *The Why.*

15. Jason and Richman, "How Science Can Stigmatize."

16. Carruthers et al., "Myalgic Encephalomyelitis."

17. Buchwald et al., "A Chronic Illness Characterized by Fatigue."

18. Ware, "Suffering and the Social Construction of Illness"; Ware, "Society, Mind and Body in Chronic Fatigue Syndrome."

19. Ware, "Society, Mind and Body in Chronic Fatigue Syndrome."

20. Iskander, "Interview with Dr. Anthony Komaroff."

21. Young, *The Harmony of Illusions*; Hacking, *Rewriting the Soul.*

22. Nichter, "Idioms of Distress Revisited."

23. Kleinman and Kleinman, "How Bodies Remember."

24. Kleinman and Kleinman, "How Bodies Remember," 713–15.

25. Kleinman, "Neurasthenia and Depression"; Kleinman, *Social Origins of Distress and Disease*; Kleinman, "Pain and Resistance"; Kleinman, *Illness Narratives.*

26. Nichter, "Idioms of Distress Revisited."

27. Kleinman, *Rethinking Psychiatry.*

28. Kleinman, *Rethinking Psychiatry,* 7.

29. Kleinman, *Rethinking Psychiatry,* 7. Although neurasthenia had been removed from the third iteration of the *Diagnostic and Statistical Manual* (DSM), it was added back to the DSM-IV in 1994 in the "Glossary of Cultural-Bound Syndromes" section, listed as *shenjing shuairuo,* based on Kleinman's influential research.

30. Kleinman and Kleinman, "How Bodies Remember," 715.

31. Lee, "The Vicissitudes of Neurasthenia in Chinese Societies."

32. Kleinman, *Writing at the Margin,* 38.

33. Kleinman, *Writing at the Margin,* 38.

34. Kleinman, *Writing at the Margin,* 38. Refer to *Writing at the Margin* for a more in-depth review of Kleinman's writing on vitality.

35. Kleinman and Kleinman, "How Bodies Remember," 716.

36. Langer, *Holocaust Testimonies*, 6, quoted in Kleinman and Kleinman, "How Bodies Remember," 117.

37. Langer, *Holocaust Testimonies*, 35.

38. Lee, "Diagnosis Postponed."

39. Foucault, *Power and Knowledge*; Young, *The Harmony of Illusions*.

40. Lee, "Diagnosis Postponed," 352.

41. Lee and Kleinman, "Are Somatoform Disorders Changing with Time?"

42. Kleinman, *Social Origins of Distress and Disease*; Kleinman and Kleinman, "How Bodies Remember."

43. Kleinman, *Social Origins of Distress and Disease*, 164–66.

44. Kleinman, *Writing at the Margin*, 36–40.

45. Lee, "Diagnosis Postponed," 353.

46. Lee, "Diagnosis Postponed," 352–56.

47. Zhang, *Anxious China*.

48. Kleinman and Straus, "Introduction."

49. Bock and Whelan, *Ciba Foundation Symposium 173*, 1.

50. Zheng et al., "Neurasthenia in Chinese Students and Visiting Scholars in the United States."

51. Kleinman, *Rethinking Psychiatry*; Kohrt et al., "Cultural Concepts of Distress and Psychiatric Disorders."

52. Kleinman and Straus, "Introduction," 3.

53. Kleinman and Straus, "Introduction," 3.

54. Shorter, "Chronic Fatigue in Historical Perspective."

55. Shorter, *From Paralysis to Fatigue*, 221.

56. Kleinman and Straus, "Introduction," 40.

57. Kleinman and Straus, "Introduction," 38.

58. Ware, "Society, Mind and Body in Chronic Fatigue Syndrome," 71.

59. Ware and Kleinman, "Culture and Somatic Experience."

60. This summary of events involved a combination of close reading of Hillary Johnson's work, including *The Why*, as well as interviews with Arthur Kleinman, Anthony Fauci, and Emily Lim Rogers. Fauci explained how NIAID at the time was swept up in HIV/AIDS research and little breath was available to focus on other health conditions, particularly ones that disabled patients (especially women) severely (as opposed to causing imminent death).

61. Fukuda et al., "The Chronic Fatigue Syndrome."

62. Carruthers et al., "Myalgic Encephalomyelitis."

63. Jason et al., "The Development of a Revised Canadian Myalgic Encephalomyelitis Chronic Fatigue Syndrome Case Definition."

64. Carruthers et al., "Myalgic Encephalomyelitis."

65. Seligman, "Learned Helplessness."

66. Miller and Seligman, "Depression and Learned Helplessness in Man."

67. Wessely and Powell, "Fatigue Syndromes."

68. Butler et al., "Cognitive Behaviour Therapy in Chronic Fatigue Syndrome"; Abel, *Sick and Tired*, 128–29.

69. Butler et al., "Cognitive Behaviour Therapy in Chronic Fatigue Syndrome"; Abel, *Sick and Tired*, 128–29.

70. Butler et al., "Cognitive Behaviour Therapy in Chronic Fatigue Syndrome"; Abel, *Sick and Tired*, 128–29.

71. Wessely, "The Neuropsychiatry of Chronic Fatigue Syndrome," 208.

72. Tuller, "Worse Than Disease: Curing Chronic Fatigue."

73. Wessely and Cleare, "Chronic Fatigue Syndrome," 460–66.

74. Butler et al., "Cognitive Behaviour Therapy in Chronic Fatigue Syndrome."

75. Cleare, "The Neuroendocrinology of Chronic Fatigue Syndrome."

76. Sharpe and Wessely, "Putting the Rest Cure to Rest—Again."

77. Sharpe, "Psychiatric Management of PVFS."

78. The principal investigators of the PACE Trial were Trudie Chalder, a professor of CVT in the Department of Psychological Medicine at King's College, London; Michael Sharpe, a professor of psychological medicine in the Department of Psychiatry at the University of Oxford; and Peter D. White, an emeritus professor of psychological medicine at Queen Mary College, London.

79. Abel, *Sick and Tired*, 129; Burgess and Chalder, *PACE Manuel for Participants*, 12.

80. White et al., "Comparison of Adaptive Pacing Therapy."

81. White et al., "Recovery from Chronic Fatigue Syndrome after Treatments Given in the PACE Trial."

82. Bithell, "Review of the First Three Years of the Mental Health Research Function at the Science Media Centre."

83. Gallagher, "Chronic Fatigue Syndrome."

84. Tuller, "Trial by Error: Open Letter to The Lancet, Version 3.0"; Davis et al., "An Open Letter to Dr Richard Horton and The Lancet."

85. Clayton, "Beyond Myalgic Encephalomyelitis."

86. Bernstein, "Chronic Fatigue Syndrome Is a Physical Disorder."

87. O'Rourke, "A New Name, and Wider Recognition, for Chronic Fatigue Syndrome," quoted in Abel, *Sick and Tired*, 131.

88. O'Rourke, "A New Name, and Wider Recognition, for Chronic Fatigue Syndrome"; Rehmeyer and Tuller, "Getting It Wrong on Chronic Fatigue Syndrome"; Khazan, "The Tragic Neglect of Chronic Fatigue Syndrome."

89. Wadman, "NIH to Double Funding for Chronic Fatigue Syndrome," quoted in Abel, *Sick and Tired*, 131.

90. Tuller, "Trial by Error"; Geraghty, "PACE-gate."

91. Tuller, "Trial by Error: The Troubling Case of the PACE Chronic Fatigue Syndrome Study," summary.

92. Tuller, "An Open Letter to The Lancet, Again."

93. Tuller, "Reexamining Chronic Fatigue Syndrome Research and Treatment Policy."

94. Geraghty, "PACE-gate"; Tuller, "Trial by Error: Open Letter to The Lancet, Version 3.0."

95. Tuller, "Trial by Error: Open Letter to The Lancet, Version 3.0"; Clayton, "Beyond Myalgic Encephalomyelitis."

96. The governmental review of the PACE Trial is spelled out in this Health Research Authority correspondence by Sir Jonathan Montgomery regarding the PACE Trial review on 29 January 2019: https://www.parliament.uk/globalassets/documents/commons-committees/science-technology/Correspondence/190129-Sir-Jonathan-Montgomery-Health-Research-Authority-to-Chair-re-PACE-trial.pdf

CHAPTER THREE

1. Murray, *The Widening Circle*; Singer, *Anthropology of Infectious Disease*, 114.

2. Steere et al., "The Emergence of Lyme Disease."

3. Rawls, *Unlocking Lyme*.

4. Keller et al., "New Insights into the Tyrolean Iceman's Origin and Phenotype as Inferred by Whole-Genome Sequencing," referenced in Davis and Nichter, "The Lyme Wars."

5. Parthasarathy et al., "The FGF/FGFR System in the Microglial Neuroinflammation with *Borrelia burgdorferi*."

6. Horowitz, *Why Can't I Get Better?*

7. Auwaerter et al., "Antiscience and Ethical Concerns Associated with Advocacy of Lyme Disease." For a critique: Dumes, "Paradise Poisoned."

8. Refer to a few key texts: Dumes, *Divided Bodies*; Rawls, *Unlocking Lyme*.

9. Hunt et al., "Racial Differences in the Diagnosis of Lyme Disease in Children."

10. Fagen et al., "Medical Gaslighting and Lyme Disease."

11. Dumes, *Divided Bodies*.

12. O'Rourke, *The Invisible Kingdom*, 104.

13. Dumit, "When Explanations Rest"; Dumit, "Illnesses You Have to Fight to Get."

14. Dumit, "When Explanations Rest"; Dumit, "Illnesses You Have to Fight to Get."

15. Horowitz, *Why Can't I Get Better?*

16. Dumit, "Illnesses You Have to Fight to Get."

17. Dumes, *Divided Bodies*, 7.

18. Davis and Nichter, "The Lyme Wars."

19. Cleghorn, *Unwell Women*.

20. Dumes, *Divided Bodies*, 118.

21. Dumes, *Divided Bodies*, 165. Many scholars have referred to this as the Lyme wars: Davis and Nichter, "The Lyme Wars"; Stricker and Johnson, "The Lyme Disease Chronicles, Continued"; Tonks, "Lyme Wars"; Weintraub, *Cure Unknown*.

22. Dumes, *Divided Bodies*; Spielman et al., "Institutional Responses to the Emergence of Lyme Disease and Its Companion Infections in North America."

23. Davis and Nichter, "The Lyme Wars"; Dumes, *Divided Bodies*.

24. Dumes, "Lyme Disease and the Epistemic Tensions of 'Medically Unexplained Illnesses.'"

25. Dumes, *Divided Bodies*.

26. Davis and Nichter, "The Lyme Wars."

27. O'Rourke, *The Invisible Kingdom*, 198; Dumes, *Divided Bodies*, 62.

28. Lantos et al., "AAN/ACR/IDSA 2020 Guidelines for the Prevention, Diagnosis and Treatment of Lyme Disease."

29. Aronowitz, "Lyme Disease"; Davis and Nichter, "The Lyme Wars."

30. O'Rourke, *The Invisible Kingdom*, 198.

31. Dumes, *Divided Bodies*, 190–91, quoted in Timmermans and Berg, *The Gold Standard*.

32. Kruse and Vassar, "Unbreakable?"; Adams, *Metrics*.

33. Dumes, *Divided Bodies*, 197.

34. Davis and Nichter, "The Lyme Wars."

35. Dumes, *Divided Bodies*, 197.

36. Dumes, *Divided Bodies*, 213.

37. Dumit, "Illnesses You Have to Fight to Get," 578.

38. Dumit, "Illnesses You Have to Fight to Get."

39. Dumes, *Divided Bodies*, 152.

40. Kenworthy, *Crowded Out*.

CHAPTER FOUR

1. Sontag, *Illness as Metaphor and AIDS and Its Metaphors*.

2. Greenhalgh, *Under the Medical Gaze*.

3. Grounding articles for weathering (Geronimus), allostatic load (McEwen), and neuroexposomes (Heffernan and Hare) are listed here for further reading; they express ideas of cumulative insults from various sources building throughout the body and across the life course and pushing bodies/people over thresholds into sickness: Geronimus, "The Weathering Hypothesis and the Health of African American Women and Infants"; McEwen, "Stress, Adaptation, and Disease"; Heffernan and Hare, "Tracing Environmental Exposure from Neurodevelopment to Neurodegeneration."

4. Sapolsky, *Why Zebra's Don't Get Ulcers*, 13–14.

5. Sapolsky, *Why Zebra's Don't Get Ulcers*.

6. Greenhalgh, *Under the Medical Gaze*.

7. For a long analysis of eating disorders in America, see Lester, *Famished*.

8. Cleghorn, *Unwell Women*, 237; Nezhat et al., "Endometriosis."

9. Cleghorn, *Unwell Women*, 237; Sampson, "Peritoneal Endometriosis Due to the Menstrual Dissemination of Endometriosis into the Peritoneal Cavity."

10. Cleghorn, *Unwell Women*, 237; Holmes, "Endometriosis."

11. Hadler, "If You Have to Prove You Are Ill, You Can't Get Well."

12. Hadler, "If You Have to Prove You Are Ill, You Can't Get Well," 2398.

13. Hadler, "If You Have to Prove You Are Ill, You Can't Get Well," 2399.

14. Dumes, *Divided Bodies*, 160.

15. Barnes, *Health Problems*, 103.

16. Van der Kolk, *The Body Keeps the Score*.

17. Ginsburg and Rapp, *Disability Worlds*, 56–57.

18. Wilson, *Gut Feminism*, 59–63.

19. Lester, *Famished*, 37–39.

20. Wilson, *Gut Feminism*, 65–66.

21. Lester, *Famished*, 59.

22. Felitti et al., "Relationship of Childhood Abuse and Household Dysfunction to Many of the Leading Causes of Death in Adults."

23. Whitaker et al., "The Interaction of Adverse Childhood Experiences and Gender as Risk Factors for Depression and Anxiety Disorders in US Adults."

24. Veyrié et al., "Endometriosis and Pregnancy."

25. Merz et al., "Pregnancy and Autoimmune Disease."

26. National Cancer Institutes, "Mast Cell," https://www.cancer.gov /publications/dictionaries/cancer-terms/def/mast-cell Accessed March 22, 2024.

27. Zanza et al., "Cytokine Storm in COVID-19."

28. Carter et al., "Mastocytosis."

29. Taylor, *Disabled Ecologies*, 31.

30. Wilson, *Gut Feminism*, 65–67.

31. Wilson, *Psychosomatic*, 22–24.

32. Yong, *I Contain Multitudes*.

33. Alaimo, *Bodily Natures*; Taylor, *Disabled Ecologies*.

34. Ailioaie et al., "Gut Microbiota and Mitochondria."

35. McEwen, "Stress, Adaptation, and Disease."

36. Vojdani et al., "Persistent SARS-CoV-2 Infection, EBV, HHV-6 and Other Factors May Contribute to Inflammation and Autoimmunity in Long COVID."

37. Prior, *Forgotten Plague*, documentary film with interview with Mike VanElzakker, minute 50–52.

38. VanElzakker, "Chronic Fatigue Syndrome from Vagus Nerve Infection."

39. VanElzakker, "Chronic Fatigue Syndrome from Vagus Nerve Infection."

40. Dani et al., "Autonomic Dysfunction in 'Long COVID.'" Amy Proal has several interviews online that are worth listening to, such as *PolyBio's Dr. Amy Proal: Transforming Diagnosis and Treatment of Complex Chronic Inflammatory Conditions*, https://polybio.org/presentations/polybios-dr-amy-proal-transforming-diagnosis-treatment-of-complex-chronic-inflammatory-conditions/.

41. Lladós et al., "Vagus Nerve Dysfunction in the Post-COVID-19 Condition."

42. Davis et al., "Long COVID: Major Findings, Mechanisms and Recommendations."

43. Del Carpio-Orantes, "Etiopathogenic Theories about Long COVID."

44. Ailioaie et al., "Gut Microbiota and Mitochondria."

45. Ramanujan, "Immune T Cells Become Exhausted in Chronic Fatigue Syndrome Patients."

46. Iu et al., "Transcriptional Reprogramming Primes CD8+ T Cells toward Exhaustion in Myalgic Encephalomyelitis/Chronic Fatigue Syndrome."

47. Davis et al., "Long COVID: Major Findings, Mechanisms and Recommendations."

CHAPTER FIVE

1. Wang et al., "Associations of Depression, Anxiety, Worry, Perceived Stress, and Loneliness Prior to Infection with Risk of Post–COVID-19 Conditions."

2. Sapolsky, *Why Zebras Don't Get Ulcers*.

3. Hay, "Suffering in a Productive World"; Ware, "Toward a Model of Social Course in Chronic Illness"; Lewis, "A Working Definition of Ableism."

4. King, *STET, Damnit! The Misanthrope's Corner, 1991–2002*.

5. Myers, *Breaking Points*, 8–15.

6. Yong, "Reporting on Long Covid Taught Me to Be a Better Journalist."

7. Becker et al., "Assessment of Cognitive Function in Patients After COVID-19 Infection."

8. Bungenberg et al., "Long COVID-19."

9. Rogers, "Staying (at Home) with Brain Fog."

10. Perlis et al., "Prevalence and Correlates of Long COVID Symptoms among US Adults."

11. Tampa et al., "Brief History of Syphilis."

12. Manly et al., "Estimating the Prevalence of Dementia and Mild Cognitive Impairment in the US."

13. Levine et al., "Virus Exposure and Neurodegenerative Disease Risk across National Biobanks."

14. Jackson, *Clearing the Fog.*

15. Premraj et al., "Mid and Long-Term Neurological and Neuropsychiatric Manifestations of Post-COVID-19 Syndrome"; van der Feltz-Cornelis et al., "Prevalence of Mental Health Conditions and Brain Fog in People with Long COVID."

16. Ginsburg and Rapp, "Disability Worlds."

17. Brea, *Unrest.*

18. Refer to Ginsburg and Rapp, *Disability Worlds.*

19. Hsu, "Why Psychological Explanations for Long COVID Are Dangerous."

20. Hsu, "The Imperative of Lived Experience for ME/CFS and Long COVID Research." The contents of this article were first delivered as a lecture at the National Institutes of Health meeting: Advancing ME/CFS Research: Identifying Targets for Intervention and Learning from Long COVID, December 12–13, 2023.

21. Hsu, "A Woman Began Screaming and Filming Me in a Parking Lot—But That's Not Even the Worst Part."

22. Hsu, "A Woman Began Screaming and Filming Me in a Parking Lot."

23. Ginsburg and Rapp, *Disability Worlds.*

24. Yoon et al., "The Demographic Features of Fatigue in the General Population Worldwide."

25. Yoon et al., "The Demographic Features of Fatigue in the General Population Worldwide."

26. Rosenthal et al., "Fatigue: An Overview."

27. Miserandino, "The Spoon Theory."

28. Hulme, "Long COVID—A Public Health Crisis Taking Out Women at the Height of Their Lives."

CHAPTER SIX

1. Wendell, *The Rejected Body*, discussed in Diedrich, "Illness (In)action."

2. Refer to Ginsburg and Rapp, "Disability Worlds," 54; also, Ginsburg and Rapp, *Disability Worlds.*

3. Dorfman, "[Un]Usual Suspects."

4. Berne et al., "Ten Principles of Disability Justice"; Mingus, "Access Intimacy."

5. Sins Invalid, "An Unshamed Claim to Beauty in the Face of Invisibility"; Sins Invalid, *Skin, Tooth, and Bone.*

6. Raffety, *From Inclusion to Justice.*

7. Brown et al., "Embodied Health Movements."

8. NBC's earliest reports on AIDS—1982. On June 17, 1982, Robert Bazell reported on a new form of "cancer" that seemed to be only affecting homosexual men. The report is described in Cook and Colby, "The Mass-Mediated Epidemic," 93.

9. NBC's earliest reports on AIDS—1982. On June 17, 1982, Robert Bazell reported on a new form of "cancer" that seemed to be only affecting homosexual men. The report is described in Cook and Colby, "The Mass-Mediated Epidemic," 93.

10. Epstein, *Impure Science*, 45–48. Reports cited: *"Pneumocystis* Pneumonia—Los Angeles," *MMWR*; "Kaposi's Sarcoma and Pneumocystis Pneumonia among Homosexual Men—New York City and California," *MMWR*; Altman, "Rare Cancer Seen in 41 Homosexuals," *The New York Times.*

11. Epstein, *Impure Science*, 49–50.

12. Packard et al., "Introduction / Emerging Illnesses as Social Process."

13. Epstein, *Impure Science*, 50.

14. Epstein, *Impure Science*, 31, 52. Murray and Payne, "The Social Classification of AIDS in American Epidemiology," 23–36.

15. Epstein, *Impure Science*, 53.

16. Epstein, *Impure Science*, 54; Bronski, "AIDing Our Guilt and Fear."

17. Epstein, *Impure Science*, 54.

18. Epstein, *Impure Science.*

19. Epstein, *Impure Science*; JD Davids, personal communication.

20. Epstein, *Impure Science*, 8.

21. France, *How to Survive a Plague.*

22. Epstein, *Impure Science*; Rogers, "Recursive Debility."

23. Centers for Disease Control and Prevention. *What Is ME/CFS?* Available at https://acrobat.adobe.com/id/urn:aaid:sc:US:73d938c6-9c1a-4d34-b28f-674410ea63cf.

24. Rogers, "Recursive Debility," 414.

25. Rogers, "Recursive Debility."

26. Rogers, "Illness, Endurance, and Proximities of AIDS Activism."

27. Epstein, *Impure Science*, 8, 348–50.

28. Gross, "Turning Disease into Political Cause"; Epstein, *Impure Science*, 348–49.

29. Ferraro, "The Anguished Politics of Breast Cancer," 26, quoted in Epstein, *Impure Science*, 348.

30. Ferraro, "The Anguished Politics of Breast Cancer," 27. See also Kolata, "Weighing Spending on Breast Cancer Research," quoted in Epstein, *Impure Science*, 348.

31. Rogers, "Illness, Endurance, and Proximities of AIDS Activism."

32. Associated Press, "Pain Meets Politics in Focus on Chronic Fatigue."

33. Hedva, "Sick Woman Theory," stanza 5.

34. Arendt, *The Human Condition*.

35. Hedva, "Sick Woman Theory," stanza 5.

36. Hedva, "Sick Woman Theory," stanza 5. The "those you love (and those you do not love)" comes from Reverend Nancy McDonald Ladd's progressive unitarian universalist teachings.

37. Hedva, "Sick Woman Theory," final stanza.

38. Hedva, "Sick Woman Theory."

39. https://me-pedia.org/wiki/Welcome_to_MEpedia.

40. Diedrich, *Illness Politics and Hashtag Activism*.

41. #MillionsMissing website, a part of #MEAction: https://millionsmissing.meaction.net/mm24/.

42. #MillionsMissing website, a part of #MEAction: http://millionsmissing.meaction.net.

43. Davids and Khanna, "Such a Powerful Love," 235.

44. Davids and Khanna, "Such a Powerful Love," 235.

45. Davids and Khanna, "Such a Powerful Love," 238.

46. O'Brien et al., "Exploring Disability from the Perspective of Adults Living with HIV/AIDS."

47. Rogers, "The Lapsed Ethnographer"; Hedva, "Sick Woman Theory," stanza 5.

48. Raffety and Worrall, "Yo-Yo Hope, 'Symptom Talk,' and the Courage *Not* to Be Well."

49. This quote builds on Dorfman's work on identity and disability, such as Dorfman, "Re-Claiming Disability," 197–98, 204. Dorfman has been writing on long COVID disability extensively: Dorfman, "Pandemic 'Disability Cons'"; Raz and Dorfman, "Bans on COVID-19 Mask Requirements vs Disability Accommodations"; Dorfman, "Experimental Jurisprudence of Health and Disability Law."

50. Dorfman, "Fear of the Disability Con."

51. O'Brien et al., "Exploring Disability from the Perspective of Adults Living with HIV/AIDS."

52. Perego et al., "Why the Patient-Made Term 'Long Covid' Is Needed"; Prior, *The Long Haul*; Mendenhall, "Long COVID and the Rise of Digital Patient Activism."

53. Lowenstein, "We Need to Talk about What Coronavirus Recoveries Look like."

54. https://www.wearebodypolitic.com/about-body-politic

55. https://www.wearebodypolitic.com/covid-19

56. Basu, "Covid-19 'Long Haulers' Are Organizing Online to Study Themselves"; https://www.longcovidsos.org/; https://patientresearchcovid19.com/.

57. Patient-Led Research Collaborative. "Report: What Does COVID-19 Recovery Actually Look Like?" https://patientresearchcovid19.com/research/report-1/.

58. Davis et al., "Characterizing Long COVID in an International Cohort."

59. They were funded by small grants from Patient-Centered Outcomes Research Institute, or PCORI, and a large donation from crypto mogul Vitalik Buterin. Although, PLRC is struggling financially now.

60. https://patientresearchcovid19.com/patient-generated-hypotheses-issue-may-2023/.

61. Prior, *The Long Haul*. https://www.longhauler-advocacy.org/.

62. Prior, *The Long Haul*, 75.

63. Proal and VanElzakker, "Long COVID or Post-Acute Sequelae of COVID-19 (PASC)."

64. Prior, *The Long Haul*, 127.

65. Prior, *The Long Haul*.

66. Barbarin, "The Pandemic Tried to Break Me, but I Know My Black Disabled Life Is Worthy."

67. Navarro, "Black and Unbelieved."

68. Chimére wrote a letter, entitled "Dear Black women: A Letter to My Sisters with Long Covid," describing her devotion to bringing together Black women living with long COVID. She wrote: "Writing you this letter is not how I imagined we would meet. But three years ago, when death echoed its hollow voice in the chambers of my body, I thought of you, and knew you would need this kind of love, too. The kind that sits next to you with no judgment as you try to make sense—on the days you can—of what Covid-19 is doing to your body. Love that is unbeholden to what you do, how you look, or how the world treats you. This love is wrapped in familiarity and protection. It arrives with a keen awareness of your struggle. I am you. And I, too, am living with what you are living through. Together, we are Black women living with Long Covid."

CHAPTER SEVEN

1. Learn more about Ty Godwin's journey on his blog, https://www.seekingbostonmarathon.com/.

2. Hales et al., "Prescription Drug Use among Adults Aged 40–79 in the United States and Canada"; National Institutes of Health, "The Dangers of Polypharmacy and the Case for Deprescribing in Older Adults."

3. Mulligan and Castañeda, *Unequal Coverage*.

4. Kenworthy, *Crowded Out*.

5. Kenworthy, *Crowded Out*, 51.

6. Carruth et al., "Structural Vulnerability."

7. Holmes, *Fresh Fruit, Broken Bodies*, 125.

8. Dumit, "Illnesses You Have to Fight to Get."

9. Bogart et al., "COVID-19 Related Medical Mistrust, Health Impacts, and Potential Vaccine Hesitancy among Black Americans Living with HIV."

10. Fricker, *Epistemic Injustice*, 1.

11. Fricker, *Epistemic Injustice*, 17.

12. Thinking about epistemic injustice in these terms was suggested first by Jen Fricas, a nursing and public health professor, who has lived with ME/CFS for several years.

13. Fricker, *Epistemic Injustice*, 17.

14. Fricker, *Epistemic Injustice*, 17.

15. Fricker, *Epistemic Injustice*, 18.

16. Crenshaw, "Demarginalizing the Intersection of Race and Sex," 139. Intersectionality is a bedrock of intellectual framing for many Black feminist health scholars such as Whitney Pirtle, Hanna Garth, and Ashanté Reese; one good resource is to look through the Cite Black Women collective: https://www.citeblackwomencollective.org/our-collective.html.

17. Pryma, "Even My Sister Says I'm Acting Like a Crazy to Get a Check."

18. Hulisz, "Amyotrophic Lateral Sclerosis."

19. There is emerging evidence of familial ALS too: https://blackdoctor.org/living-with-als-stephen-frays-inspiring-path-to-awareness/.

20. Carter, "The 'Truth' about ALS"; Carter, "The Racial Thinking behind ALS diagnosis."

21. Carter, "The 'Truth' about ALS."

22. Canada and Carter, "Weathering Anti-Blackness"; Carter, "Gaslighting."

23. Pons-Estel et al., "Understanding the Epidemiology and Progression of Systemic Lupus Erythematosus"; Manzi et al., "Age-Specific Incidence Rates of MI and Angina in Women with SLE."

24. Chae et al., "Racial Discrimination, Disease Activity, and Organ Damage"; Angum et al., "The Prevalence of Autoimmune Disorders in Women with SLE"; Roberts and Erdei, "Comparative United States Autoimmune Disease Rates for 2010–2016 by Sex, Geographic Region, and Race."

25. Barbarin, "The Pandemic Tried to Break Me, but I Know My Black Disabled Life Is Worthy."

26. Hatfield-Timajchy, *Delayed Diagnosis*.

27. Frank, *The Wounded Storyteller*.

28. Smith, "Doctors Didn't Believe That I Had COVID-19. I Found a Way to Make Them Listen."

29. Hsu et al., "Patients as Knowledge Partners in the Context of Complex Chronic Conditions," 4.

30. Aronowitz, "When Do Symptoms Become a Disease?" 803–8.

CHAPTER EIGHT

1. Atlanta Journal Constitution, "A Look at Alana Shepherd of Atlanta's Shepherd Center." https://appnews.ajc.com/QVDNYTO4EBET7O6KSR6BRYVXLI /content.html.

2. Men are more likely to experience spinal injuries than women: Shackelford et al., "A Comparison of Women and Men with Spinal Cord Injury."

3. Ginsburg and Rapp, *Disability Worlds*, 28.

4. Hedva, "Sick Woman Theory," 2.

5. Wahlberg, "Serious Disease as Kinds of Living"; Manderson and Wahlberg, "Chronic Living in a Communicable World"; Manderson et al., *Viral Loads*.

6. Becker, *Disrupted Lives*; Van der Kolk, *The Body Keeps the Score*.

7. Galanis et al., "Nurses' Burnout and Associated Risk Factors during the COVID-19 Pandemic."

8. Lowe et al., "Structural Discrimination in Pandemic Policy."

9. Rivera-Núñez et al., "Experiences of Black and Latinx Health Care Workers in Support Roles during the COVID-19 Pandemic."

10. Snowden and Snowden, "Coronavirus Trauma and African Americans' Mental Health."

11. Fahs, "Fat and Furious."

12. Jackson, *Clearing the Fog*.

CONCLUSION

1. Stetson, "The Yellow Wallpaper."

2. *Septad* was coined by Ilene Ruhoy, a neurologist at Mount Sinai South in Oceanside, New York. https://spinalcsfleak.org/dr-ilene-ruhoy-complex-patient/.

3. Hsu et al., "Patients as Knowledge Partners in the Context of Complex Chronic Conditions," 4.

Bibliography

"160 Victims at Lake Tahoe: Chronic Flu-Like Illness a Medical Mystery Story." *Los Angeles Times*, June 7, 1986. https://www.latimes.com/archives/la-xpm-1986-06-07-mn-9956-story.html.

Abel, Emily. *Sick and Tired: An Intimate Story of Fatigue*. University of North Carolina Press, 2021.

Adams, Vincanne. *Metrics: What Counts in Global Health*. Duke University Press, 2016.

Ailioaie, Laura Marinela, Constantin Ailioaie, and Gerhard Litscher. "Gut Microbiota and Mitochondria: Health and Pathophysiological Aspects of Long COVID." *International Journal of Molecular Sciences* 24, no. 24 (2023): 17198.

Alaimo, Stacy. *Bodily Natures: Science, Environment, and the Material Self*. Indiana University Press, 2010.

Allbutt, Clifford. "Nervous Diseases and Modern Life." *Contemporary Review* 67 (1895): 210–31.

Angum, Fariha, Tahir Khan, Jasndeep Kaler, Lena Siddiqui, and Azhar Hussain. "The Prevalence of Autoimmune Disorders in Women: A Narrative Review." *Cureus* 12, no. 5 (2020): e8094.

Arendt, Hannah. *The Human Condition.* University of Chicago Press, 1958.

Aronowitz, Robert. "From Myalgic Encephalitic to Yuppie Flu." In *Framing Disease: Studies in Cultural History,* edited by Robert Aronowitz. Rutgers University Press, 1992.

———. "Lyme Disease: The Social Construction of a New Disease and Its Social Consequences." *Millbank Quarterly* 69, no. 1 (1991): 79–112.

———. "When Do Symptoms Become a Disease?" *Annals of Internal Medicine* 134, no. 9 Pt. 2 (2001): 803–8.

Associated Press. "Pain Meets Politics in Focus on Chronic Fatigue." NBC News, February 18, 2007. https://www.nbcnews.com/health/health-news/pain-meets-politics-focus-chronic-fatigue-flna1c9470207.

Auwaerter, Paul G., Johan S. Bakken, Raymond Dattwyler, Stephen Dumerl, John Halerin, Edward McSweegan, Robert Nadelman, et al. "Antiscience and Ethical Concerns Associated with Advocacy of Lyme Disease." *Lancet Infectious Disease* 11, no. 9 (2011): 713–19.

Barbarin, Imani. "The Pandemic Tried to Break Me, but I Know My Black Disabled Life Is Worthy." *Cosmopolitan,* March 11, 2022. https://www.cosmopolitan.com/entertainment/a39355245/imani-barbarin-black-disabled-activist-self-love/.

Barnes, Elizabeth. *Health Problems.* Cambridge University Press, 2023.

———. *The Minority Body.* Cambridge University Press, 2016.

Barry, John. *The Great Influenza: The Story of the Deadliest Pandemic in History.* Penguin Books, 2005.

Basu, Tanya. "Covid-19 'Long Haulers' Are Organizing Online to Study Themselves." *MIT Technology Review,* August 12, 2020. https://www.technologyreview.com/2020/08/12/1006602/covid-19-long-haulers-are-organizing-online-to-study-themselves/.

Beard, George. *American Nervousness: Its Causes and Consequences (A Supplement to Nervous Exhaustion, Neurasthenia).* G. P. Putnam's Sons, 1881.

———. "Neurasthenia, or Nervous Exhaustion." *Boston Medical and Surgical Journal* 80, no. 13 (1869): 217–21.

———. *A Practical Treatise on Nervous Exhaustion (Neurasthenia): Its Symptoms, Nature, Sequences, Treatment,* edited with notes and additions by A. D. Rockwell. The Publishers Printing Company, 1880.

Becker, Gay. *Disrupted Lives: How People Create Meaning in a Chaotic World.* University of California Press, 1999.

Becker, Jacqueline H., Jenny J. Lin, Molly Doernberg, Kimberly Stone, Allison Navis, Joanne R. Festa, and Juan P. Wisnivesky. "Assessment of Cognitive Function in Patients After COVID-19 Infection." *JAMA Network Open* 4, no. 10 (2021): e2130645.

Berne, Patricia, Aurora Levins Morales, David Langstaff, and Sins Invalid. "Ten Principles of Disability Justice." *WSQ: Women's Studies Quarterly* 46, no. 1 & 2 (2018): 227–30.

Bernstein, Lenny. "Chronic Fatigue Syndrome Is a Physical Disorder, Not a Psychological Illness, Panel Says." *Washington Post*, February 10, 2015. https://www.washingtonpost.com/news/to-your-health/wp/2015/02/10/chronic-fatigue-syndrome-is-a-real-condition-not-a-psychological-illness-expert-panel-says/.

Bithell, Claire. *Review of the First Three Years of the Mental Health Research Function at the Science Media Centre.* Science Media Center (Report), February, 2013. https://www.sciencemediacentre.org/uploads/2013/03/Review-of-the-first-three-years-of-the-mental-health-research-function-at-the-Science-Media-Centre.pdf.

Blattner, R.J. "Benign Myalgic Encephalomyelitis (Akureyri Disease, Iceland Disease)." *Journal of Pediatrics* 49, no. 4 (1956): 504–6.

Bock, Gregory R., and Julie Whelan, Eds. *Ciba Foundation Symposium 173—Chronic Fatigue Syndrome.* (Ciba Foundation 1993.) Novartis Foundation Symposia, 2007.

Bogart, Laura M., Bisola O. Ojikutu, Keshav Tyagi, David J. Klein, Matt G. Mutchler, Lu Dong, Sean J. Lawrence, Damone R. Thomas, and Sarah Kellman. "COVID-19 Related Medical Mistrust, Health Impacts, and Potential Vaccine Hesitancy among Black Americans Living with HIV." *Journal of Acquired Immune Deficiency Syndrome* 86, no. 2 (2021): 200–207.

Brea, Jennifer. *Unrest.* 2017. https://www.youtube.com/watch?v=XOpyLTyVxco&t=2905s.

Breuer, Josef, and Sigmond Freud. *Studies on Hysteria (German: Studien über Hysterie).* Basic Books, 1895.

Brigo, F. "Jean-Martin Charcot (1825–1893) and His Second Thoughts about Hysteria." *Arquivos de Neuro-Psiquiatria* 79, no. 2 (2021): 173–74.

Bronski, Michael. "AIDing Our Guilt and Fear." *Gay Community News*, October 9, 1982, 8.

Brown, Phil, Stephen Zavestoski, Sabrina McCormick, Brian Mayer, Rachel Morello-Frosch, and Rebecca Gasior Altman. "Embodied Health Movements: New Approaches to Social Movements in Health." *Sociology of Health and Illness* 26, no. 1 (2004): 55–80.

Bruno, Richard L., Susan J. Creange, and Nancy M. Frick. "Parallels between Post-Polio Fatigue and Chronic Fatigue Syndrome: A Common Pathophysiology?" *American Journal of Medicine* 105, no. 3 Suppl. 1 (1998): 66S–73S.

Buchwald, Dedra, Paul R. Cheney, Daniel L. Peterson, Berch Henry, Susan B. Wormsley, Ann Geiger, Dharam V. Ablashi, et al. "A Chronic Illness Characterized by Fatigue, Neurologic and Immunologic Disorders, and Active Human Herpesvirus Type 6 Infection." *Annals of Internal Medicine* 116, no. 2 (1992): 103–13.

Bungenberg, Julia, Karen Humkamp, Christian Hohenfeld, Marcus Immanuel Rust, Ummehan Ermis, Michael Dreher, Niels-Ulrik Korbinian Hartmann, et al. "Long COVID-19: Objectifying Most Self-Reported Neurological Symptoms." *Annals of Clinical and Translational Neurology* 9, no. 2 (2022):141–54.

Burgess, Mary, and Trudie Chalder. *PACE Manuel for Participants, Cognitive Behaviour Therapy for CFS/ME*. #MEpedia, November 2004. http://www.me-pedia.org/images/7/7a/PACE-cbt-participant-manuel.pdf.

Butler, S., Trudie Chalder, M. Ron, and Simon Wessely. "Cognitive Behaviour Therapy in Chronic Fatigue Syndrome." *Journal of Neurology, Neurosurgery, and Psychiatry* 51 (1991): 153–154.

Canada, Tracie, and Chelsey R. Carter. "Weathering Anti-Blackness: Injury, Brain Trauma and Neurodegeneration in American Sport." *Current Anthropology* 65, no. 26 (2024): S177–95.

Carruth, Lauren, Carlos Martinez, Lahra Smith, Katharine Donato, Carlos Piñones-Rivera, and James Quesada. "Structural Vulnerability: Migration and Health in Social Context." *BMJ Global Health* 6 (2021): e005109.

Carruthers, Bruce M., Anil Kumar Jain, Kenny L. De Meirleir, Daniel L. Peterson, Nancy G. Klimas, A. Martin Lerner, Alison C. Bested, et al. "Myalgic Encephalomyelitis/Chronic Fatigue Syndrome: Clinical Working Case Definition, Diagnostic and Treatment Protocols." *Journal of Chronic Fatigue Syndrome* 11, no. 2 (2003): 7–115.

Carter, Chelsey. "Gaslighting: ALS, Anti-Blackness, and Medicine." *Feminist Anthropology* 3, no. 4 (2022): 243.

———. "The Racial Thinking behind ALS Diagnosis." *Anthropology News*, March 1, 2021. https://www.anthropology-news.org/articles/the-racial-thinking-behind-als-diagnosis/#citation.

———. "The 'Truth' about ALS: Reconciling Bias, Motives, and Etiological Gaps." *Somatosphere*, September 29, 2020. http://somatosphere.net/2020/als-bias-motives-etiological-gaps.html/.

Carter, Melody C., Dean D. Metcalfe, and Hirsh D. Komarow. "Mastocytosis." *Immunology and Allergy Clinics of North America* 34, no. 1 (2014): 181–96.

Chae, David H., Connor D. Martz, Thomas E. Fuller-Rowell, Erica C. Spears, Tianqi Tenchi Gao Smith, Evelyn A. Hunter, Cristina Drenkard, and S. Sam Lim. "Racial Discrimination, Disease Activity, and Organ Damage: The Black Women's Experiences Living with Lupus (BeWELL) Study." *American Journal of Epidemiology* 188, no. 8 (2019): 1434–43.

Chambers, Thomas K. "Clinical Lecture on Hysteria." *British Medical Journal* 2, no. 51 (1861): 651–55.

Charcot, Jean Martin. *Leçons du Mardi à la Salpêtrière: policliniques, 1887–1888.* Aux bureaux du Progres medical, 1887–9.

Chrichton Miller, H. *Functional Nerve Disease: An Epitome of War Experience for the Practitioner.* Henry Frowde, Hodder & Stoughton, 1920.

Cite Black Women Collective. https://www.citeblackwomencollective.org/our-collective.html.

Clayton, Ellen Wright. "Beyond Myalgic Encephalomyelitis/Chronic Fatigue Syndrome: An IOM Report on Redefining an Illness." *JAMA* 313, no. 11 (2015): 1101–2.

Cleare, Anthony J. "The Neuroendocrinology of Chronic Fatigue Syndrome." *Endocrine Reviews* 24, no. 2 (2003): 236–52.

Cleghorn, Elinor. *Unwell Women: Misdiagnosis and Myth in a Man-Made World.* Dutton, 2021.

Committee on the Diagnostic Criteria for Myalgic Encephalomyelitis/Chronic Fatigue Syndrome, Board on the Health of Select Populations, Institute of Medicine. *Beyond Myalgic Encephalomyelitis/Chronic Fatigue Syndrome: Redefining an Illness.* National Academies Press, February 10, 2015.

Cook, Timothy E, and David C. Colby. "The Mass-Mediated Epidemic: The Politics of AIDS on the Nightly Network New." In *AIDS: The Making of a Chronic Disease*, edited by Elizabeth Fee and Daniel M. Fox. University of California Press, 1981.

Crenshaw, Kimberlé W. "Demarginalizing the Intersection of Race and Sex: A Black Feminist Critique of Antidiscrimination Doctrine, Feminist Theory and Antiracist Politics." *University of Chicago Legal Forum* 139 (1989).

Dani, Melanie, Adreas Dirksen, Patricia Taraborrelli, Miriam Torocastro, Dimitrios Panagopoulos, Richard Sutton, and Phang Boon Lim. "Autonomic Dysfunction in 'Long COVID': Rationale, Physiology and Management Strategies." *Clinical Medicine* 21, no. 1 (2021): e63–e67.

Davids, J. D., and Naina Khanna. "Such a Powerful Love: Disabled and Chronically Ill People and Our Long Fight for Justice." In *The Long Covid Survival Guide*, edited by Fiona Lowenstein. The Experiment, 2022.

Davis, Dána-Ain. *Reproductive Injustice: Racism, Pregnancy, and Premature Birth.* New York University Press, 2019.

Davis, Georgia, and Mark Nichter. "The Lyme Wars: The Effects of Biocommunicability, Gender, and Epistemic Politics on Health Activation and Lyme Science." In *Diagnostic Controversy: Cultural Perspectives on Competing Knowledge in Healthcare*, edited by Carolyn Smith-Morris. Taylor and Francis, 2016.

Davis, Hannah E., Gina S. Assaf, Lisa McCorkell, Hannah Wei, Ryan J. Low, Yochai Re'em, Signe Redfield, Jared P. Austin, and Athena Akrami. "Characterizing Long COVID in an International Cohort: 7 Months of Symptoms and Their Impact." *eClinicalMedicine* 38 (2021): 101019.

Davis, Hannah E., Lisa McCorkell, Julia Moore Vogel, and Eric J. Topol. "Long COVID: Major Findings, Mechanisms and Recommendations." *Nature Reviews Microbiology* 21, no. 3 (2023): 133–46.

Davis, Ronald W., Jonathan C. W. Edwards, Leonard A. Jason, Bruce Levin, Vincent R. Racaniello, and Arthur L. Reingold. "An Open Letter to Dr Richard Horton and The Lancet". *Virology Blog*, November 13, 2015. https://virology.ws/2015/11/13/an-open-letter-to-dr-richard-horton-and-the-lancet/.

Del Carpio-Orantes, Luis. "Etiopathogenic Theories about Long COVID." *World Journal of Virology* 12, no. 3 (2023): 204–8.

Diedrich, Lisa. "Illness (In)action: CFS and #TimeforUnrest." *Literature and Medicine* 39, no. 1 (2021): 8–14.

———. *Illness Politics and Hashtag Activism.* University of Minnesota Press, 2024.

Dorfman, Doron. "Experimental Jurisprudence of Health and Disability Law." In *Cambridge Handbook of Experimental Jurisprudence*, edited by Kevin Tobia. Cambridge University Press, 2025.

———. "Fear of the Disability Con: Perceptions of Fraud and Special Rights Discourse." *Law & Society Review* 53, no. 4 (2024): 1051–91.

———. "Pandemic 'Disability Cons.'" *Journal of Law, Medicine & Ethics* 49 (2021): 401–9.

———. "Re-Claiming Disability: Identity, Procedural Justice, and the Disability Determination Process." *Law & Society* 42, no. 1 (2017): 195–231.

———. "[Un]Usual Suspects: Deservingness, Scarcity, and Disability Rights." *University of California Irvine Law Review* 10 (2020: 557.

Dumes, Abigail A. *Divided Bodies: Lyme Disease, Contested Illness, and Evidence-Based Medicine.* Duke University Press, 2020.

———. "Lyme Disease and the Epistemic Tensions of 'Medically Unexplained Illnesses.'" *Medical Anthropology* 39, no. 6 (2020): 441–56.

———. "Paradise Poisoned: Nature, Environmental Risk, and the Practice of Lyme Disease Prevention in the United States." In *A Companion to the Anthropology of Environmental Health*, edited by Merrill Singer. Wiley and Sons, 2016.

Dumit, Joseph. "Illnesses You Have to Fight to Get: Facts as Forces in Uncertain, Emergent Illnesses." *Social Science and Medicine* 62, no. 3 (2006): 577–90.

———. "When Explanations Rest: 'Good-Enough' Brain Science and the New Socio-Medical Disorders." *Living and Working with the New Medical Technologies: Intersections of Inquiry* 8 (2000): 209.

Edwards, Martin. "Hysteria." *Lancet* 374, no. 9702 (2009): P1669.

Ellison, James. "A Fierce Hunger: The Epidemic in Southwest Tanzania." In *The Spanish Influenza Pandemic of 1918–1919: New Perspectives*, edited by Howard Phillips and David Killingray. Routledge, 2003.

Epstein, Steven. *Impure Science: AIDS, Activism, and the Politics of Knowledge.* University of California Press, 1996.

Fagen, Jennifer L., Jeremy A. Shelton, and Jenna Luché-Thayer. "Medical Gaslighting and Lyme Disease: The Patient Experience." *Healthcare* (Basel) 12, no. 1 (2023): 78.

Fahs, Breanne. "Fat and Furious: Interrogating Fat Phobia and Nurturing Resistance in Medical Framings of Fat Bodies." *Women's Reproductive Health* 6, no. 4 (2019): 245–51.

FDA (Food and Drug Administration). *The Voice of the Patient: Chronic Fatigue Syndrome and Myalgic Encephalomyelitis.* Center for Drug Evaluation and Research (CDER), FDA, 2013.

Felitti, Vincent J., Robert F. Anda, Dale Nordenberg, David F. Williamson, Alison Spitz, Valerie Edwards, Mary P. Koss, and James S. Marks. "Relationship of Childhood Abuse and Household Dysfunction to Many of the Leading Causes of Death in Adults." *American Journal of Preventive Medicine* 14, no. 4 (1998): 245–58.

Ferraro, Susan. "The Anguished Politics of Breast Cancer." *New York Times Magazine*, August 15, 1993. https://www.nytimes.com/1993/08/15/magazine/the-anguished-politics-of-breast-cancer.html.

Foucault, Michel. *Power and Knowledge: Selected Interviews and Other Writings.* Pantheon, 1980.

France, David. *How to Survive a Plague: The Inside Story of How Citizens and Science Tamed AIDS.* Knopf, 2016.

Frank, Arthur. *The Wounded Storyteller: Body, Illness, and Ethics.* University of Chicago Press, 2007.

Fricker, Miranda. *Epistemic Injustice: Power and the Ethics of Knowing.* Oxford University Press, 2007.

Fukuda, Keiji, Stephen E. Straus, Ian Hickie, Michael C. Sharpe, James G. Dobbins, and Anthony Komaroff. "The Chronic Fatigue Syndrome: A Comprehensive Approach to Its Definition and Study. International Chronic Fatigue Syndrome Study Group." *Annals of Internal Medicine* 121, no. 12 (1994): 953–9.

Galanis, Petros, Irene Vraka, Despoina Fragkou, Angeliki Bilali, and Daphne Kaitelidou. "Nurses' Burnout and Associated Risk Factors during the COVID-19 Pandemic: A Systematic Review and Meta-analysis." *Journal of Advanced Nursing* 77, no. 8 (2021): 3286–3302.

Gallagher, Paul. "Chronic Fatigue Syndrome: Tribunal Orders Data from Controversial Trial to Be Released." *The i Paper*, August 19, 2016. https://inews .co.uk/news/health/tribunal-chronic-fatigue-syndrome-data-released-18748.

Geraghty, Keith. "'PACE-gate': When Clinical Trial Evidence Meets Open Data Access." *Journal of Health Psychology* 22, no. 9 (2017): 1106–12.

Geronimus, Arline T. "Black/White Differences in the Relationship of Maternal Age to Birthweight: A Population-Based Test of the Weathering Hypothesis." *Social Science and Medicine* 42, no. 4 (1996): 589–97.

———. "The Weathering Hypothesis and the Health of African American Women and Infants: Evidence and Speculations." *Ethnicity and Disease* 2 (1992): 207.

Gilliam, Alexander Gordon. *Epidemiological Study of an Epidemic, Diagnosed as Poliomyelitis, Occurring among the Personnel of the Los Angeles County General Hospital during the Summer of 1934*. US Government Printing Office, 1938.

Ginsburg, Faye, and Rayna Rapp. "Disability Worlds." *Annual Review of Anthropology* 42 (2013): 53–68.

———. *Disability Worlds*. Duke University Press, 2024.

Goetz, Christopher G. "Poor Beard!! Charcot's Internationalization of Neurasthenia, the 'American disease.'" *Neurology* 57, no. 3 (2001): 510–14.

Greenhalgh, Susan. *Under the Medical Gaze: Facts and Fictions of Chronic Pain*. University of California Press, 2001.

Greenwood, Anna. "Looking Back: The Strange History of Tropical Neurasthenia." *Psychologist*, March 18, 2011. https://www.bps.org.uk/psychologist /looking-back-strange-history-tropical-neurasthenia.

Griffith, Fracis Llewellyn. *The Petrie Papyri: Hieratic Papyri from Kahun and Gurob*. Bernard Quaritch, 1898.

Gross, Jane. "Turning Disease into Political Cause: First AIDS, and Now Breast Cancer." *New York Times*, January 7, 1991. https://www.nytimes.com/1991/01 /07/us/turning-disease-into-political-cause-first-aids-and-now-breast-cancer .html.

Hacking, Ian. *Rewriting the Soul: Multiple Personality and the Sciences of Memory*. Princeton University Press, 1995.

Hadler, Nortin M. "If You Have to Prove You Are Ill, You Can't Get Well: The Object Lesson of Fibromyalgia." *Spine* 21, no. 20 (1996): 2397–2400.

Hales, C. M., J. Servais, C. B. Martin, and D. Kohen. *Prescription Drug Use among Adults Aged 40–79 in the United States and Canada*. NCHS Data Brief, no 347. National Center for Health Statistics, 2019.

Hatfield-Timajchy, Kendra S. *Delayed Diagnosis: The Experience of Women with Systemic Lupus Erythematosus in Atlanta, Georgia*. Emory University ProQuest Dissertations Publishing (3298444), 2007.

Hay, M. Cameron. "Suffering in a Productive World: Chronic Illness, Visibility, and the Space beyond Agency. *American Ethnologist* 37, no. 2 (2010): 259–74.

Hedva, Johanna. "Sick Woman Theory." *Topical Cream* (blog), March 12, 2022. https://topicalcream.org/features/sick-woman-theory/.

Heffernan, Amy L., and Dominic J. Hare. "Tracing Environmental Exposure from Neurodevelopment to Neurodegeneration." *Trends in Neuroscience* 41, no. 8 (2018): 496–501.

Holmes, Gary P., Jonathan E. Kaplan, Nelson M. Gantz, Anthony L. Komaroff, Lawrence B. Schonberger, Stephen E. Straus, James F. Jones, et al. "Chronic Fatigue Syndrome: A Working Case Definition." *Annals of Internal Medicine* 108, no. 3 (1988): 387–89.

Holmes, Gary P., Jonathan E. Kaplan, John A. Stewart, Barbara Hunt, Paul F. Pinsky, and Lawrence B. Schonberger. "A Cluster of Patients with a Chronic Mononucleosis-Like Syndrome. Is Epstein-Barr Virus the Cause?" *JAMA* 257, no. 17 (1987): 2297–302.

Holmes, Seth. *Fresh Fruit, Broken Bodies: Migrant Farmworkers in the United States*. University of California Press, 2013.

Holmes, Walter R. "Endometriosis." *American Journal of Obstetrics and Gynecology* 43, no. 2 (1942): 263.

Honigsbaum, Mark, and Lakshmi Krishnan. "Taking Pandemic Sequelae Seriously: From the Russian Influenza to COVID-19 Long-Haulers." *Lancet* 396 (2020): 1389–91.

Horowitz, Richard I. *Why Can't I Get Better? Solving the Mystery of Lyme and Chronic Disease*. St. Martin's Press, 2013.

Hsu, Vox Jo. "The Imperative of Lived Experience for ME/CFS and Long COVID Research: What to Make of Patient Stories." *Social Science and Medicine—Mental Health* 5 (2023): 100291.

———. "Why Psychological Explanations for Long COVID Are Dangerous." *KevinMD MedPage Today's Conditions*, September 16, 2022. https://www

.kevinmd.com/2022/09/why-psychological-explanations-for-long-covid-are-dangerous.html.

———. "A Woman Began Screaming and Filming Me in a Parking Lot—But That's Not Even the Worst Part." *Huffpost*, December 27, 2022. https://www.huffpost.com/entry/woman-filmed-parking-lot-aapi-hate_n_639776d4e4b019c6962493e9?qqn.

Hsu, Vox Jo, Megan Moodie, Abigail Dumes, Emily Lim Rogers, Chelsey R. Carter, Emma Broder, Daisy Couture, Ilana Löwy, and Emily Mendenhall. "Patients as Knowledge Partners in the Context of Complex Chronic Conditions." *Medical Humanities* 51, no. 1 (2025): 34–38.

Hulisz, Darrell. "Amyotrophic Lateral Sclerosis: Disease State Overview." *American Journal of Managed Care* 24, 15 Suppl. (2018): S320–S326.

Hulme, Jennifer. "Long COVID—A Public Health Crisis Taking Out Women at the Height of Their Lives." *Healthy Debate*, May 26, 2022. https://healthydebate.ca/2022/05/topic/long-covid-crisis-women/.

Hunt, Kathryn M., Kenneth A. Michelson, Fran Balamuth, Amy D. Thompson, Michael N. Levas, Desiree N. Neville, Anupam B. Kharbanda, Laura Chapman, Lise E. Nigrovic; Pedi Lyme Net. "Racial Differences in the Diagnosis of Lyme Disease in Children." *Clinical Infectious Disease* 76, no. 6 (2023): 1129–31.

Hyde, Byron, and Sverrir Bergmann. "Akureyri Disease (Myalgic Encephalomyelitis), Forty Years Later." *Lancet* 2, no. 8621 (1988): 1191–92.

Iskander, John. "Interview with Dr. Anthony Komaroff." *CDC Public Health Ground Rounds.* Beyond the Data—Chronic Fatigue Syndrome: Advancing Research and Clinical Education. February 17, 2016. https://www.youtube.com/watch?v=hRdn4A2SGic.

Iu, David S., Jessica Maya, Luyen T. Vu, Elizabeth A. Fogarty, Adrian J. McNairn, Faraz Ahmed, Carl J. Franconi, et al. "Transcriptional Reprogramming Primes CD8+ T cells Toward Exhaustion in Myalgic Encephalomyelitis/Chronic Fatigue Syndrome." *Proceedings of the National Academy of Sciences* 121, no. 50 (2024): e2415119121.

Jackson, James C. *Clearing the Fog: From Surviving to Thriving with Long Covid—A Practical Guide.* Little, Brown Spark, 2023.

Jason, Leonard A., Meredyth Evans, Nicole Porter, Molly Brown, Abigail Brown, Jessica Hunnell, Valerie Anderson, Athena Lerch, Kenny

De Meirleir, and Fred Friedberg. "The Development of a Revised Canadian Myalgic Encephalomyelitis Chronic Fatigue Syndrome Case Definition." *American Journal of Biochemistry and Biotechnology* 6, no. 2 (2010): 120–35.

Jason, Leonard A., Cordelia Holbert, Susan Torres-Harding, and Renee R. Taylor. "Stigma and the Term Chronic Fatigue Syndrome." *Journal of Disability Policy Studies* 14, no. 4 (2004): 222–28.

Jason, Leonard A., and Judith A. Richman. "How Science Can Stigmatize: The Case of Chronic Fatigue Syndrome." *Journal of Chronic Fatigue Syndrome* 14, no. 4 (2008): 85–103.

Johnson, Hillary. *Osler's Web: Inside the Labyrinth of the Chronic Fatigue Syndrome Epidemic.* Crown, 1996.

———. *The Why: The Historic ME/CFS Call to Arms.* Basset Creek, 2009.

Kaplan, Kenton, and Emily Mendenhall. "Framing Long Covid through Patient Activism in the United States: A Qualitative Study." *Social Science and Medicine* 350 (2024): 116901.

Keller, Andreas, Angela Graefen, Markus Ball, Mark Matzas, Valesca Boisguerin, Frank Maixner, Petra Leidinger, et al. "New Insights into the Tyrolean Iceman's Origin and Phenotype as Inferred by Whole-Genome Sequencing." *Nature Communication* 3 (2012): 698.

Keller, Evelyn Fox. *Refiguring Life: Metaphors of Twentieth-Century Biology.* Columbia University Press, 1995.

Kenworthy, Nora. *Crowded Out: The True Cost of Crowdfunding Healthcare.* MIT Press, 2024.

Khazan, Olga. "The Tragic Neglect of Chronic Fatigue Syndrome." *The Atlantic*, October 8, 2015. https://www.theatlantic.com/health/archive/2015/10/chronic-fatigue-patients-push-for-an-elusive-cure/409534/.

King, Florence. *STET, Damnit! The Misanthrope's Corner, 1991–2002.* National Review, 2003.

Kirmayer, Laurence. "Beyond the 'New Cross-cultural Psychiatry': Cultural Biology, Discursive Psychology and the Ironies of Globalization." *Transcultural Psychiatry* 43, no. 126 (2006): 131.

———. "Mind and Body as Metaphors: Hidden Values in Biomedicine." In *Biomedicine Examined*, edited by Margaret Lock and Deborah Gordon. Kluwer Academic, 1988.

Kleinman, Arthur. *The Illness Narratives: Suffering, Healing, and the Human Conditions.* Basic Books, 1989.

———. "Neurasthenia and Depression: A Study of Somatization and Culture in China." *Culture, Medicine and Psychiatry* 6, no. 2 (1982): 117–89.

———. "Pain and Resistance: The Delegitimation and Relegitimation of Local Worlds." In *Pain as Human Experience: An Anthropological Perspective*, edited by Mary Jo D Good, Paul E. Brodwin, Byron J. Good, and Arthur Kleinman. University of California Press, 1992.

———. *Rethinking Psychiatry: From Cultural Category to Personal Experience.* Free Press, 1988.

———. *Social Origins of Distress and Disease.* Yale University Press, 1986.

———. *Writing at the Margin: Discourse between Anthropology and Medicine.* University of California Press, 1995.

Kleinman, Arthur, and Joan Kleinman. "How Bodies Remember: Social Memory and Bodily Experience of Criticism, Resistance, and Delegitimation following China's Cultural Revolution." *New Literary History* 25, no. 3 (1994): 707–23.

Kleinman, Arthur, and Stephen Straus. "Introduction." In *Ciba Foundation Symposium 173—Chronic Fatigue Syndrome*, edited by Gregory R. Bock and Julie Whelan (Ciba Foundation 1993.) Novartis Foundation Symposia, 2007.

Kohrt, Brandon A., Andrew Rasmussen, Bonnie N. Kaiser, Emily E. Haroz, Sujen M. Maharjan, Byamah B. Mutamba, Joop T. V. M. DeJong, and Devon Hinton. "Cultural Concepts of Distress and Psychiatric Disorders: Literature Review and Research Recommendations for Global Mental Health Epidemiology." *International Journal of Epidemiology* 43, no. 2 (2014): 365–406.

Kolata, Gina. "Weighing Spending on Breast Cancer Research." *New York Times*, October 20, 1993. https://www.nytimes.com/1993/10/20/health/weighing-spending-on-breast-cancer.html.

Krishnan, Lakshmi. "An Extraordinary Sequel: The 'Russian' Influenza and Enduring Sequelae in Victorian Culture." *Journal of Victorian Culture* 27, no. 2 (2022): 302–18.

Kruse, B. Chase, and B. Matt Vassar. "Unbreakable? An Analysis of the Fragility of Randomized Trials That Support Diabetes Treatment Guidelines." *Diabetes Research and Clinical Practice* 134 (2017): 91–105.

Lancet. "A New Clinical Entity?" *Lancet* 270, no. 6926 (1956): 789–90.

Langer, Lawrence. *Holocaust Testimonies.* Yale University Press, 1991.

Lantos, Paul M., Jeffrey Rumbaugh, Linda K. Bockenstedt, Yngve T. Falck-Ytter, Maria E. Aguero-Rosenfeld, Paul G. Auwaerter, Kelly Baldwin, et al. "AAN/ACR/IDSA 2020 Guidelines for the Prevention, Diagnosis and Treatment of Lyme Disease." *Clinical Infectious Diseases* 72, no. 1 (2021): e1–e48.

Latour, Bruno. *Reassembling the Social: An Introduction to Actor-Network Theory.* Oxford University Press, 2005.

Lee, Sing. "Diagnosis Postponed: Shenjing Shuairuo and the Transformation of Psychiatry in Post-Mao China." *Culture, Medicine, and Psychiatry* 23 (1999): 349–80.

———. "The Vicissitudes of Neurasthenia in Chinese Societies: Where Will It Go from the ICD-10?" *Transcultural Psychiatric Research Review* 31 (1994): 153–72.

Lee, Sing, and Arthur Kleinman. "Are Somatoform Disorders Changing with Time? The Case of Neurasthenia in China." *Psychosomatic Medicine* 69, no. 9 (2007): 846–49.

Lerner, Paul Frederick. *Hysterical Men: War, Psychiatry, and the Politics of Trauma in Germany, 1890–1930.* Cornell University Press, 2003.

Lester, Rebecca. *Famished: Eating Disorders and Failed Care in America.* University of California Press, 2019.

Levine, Kristin S., Hampton L. Leonard, Cornelis Blauwendraat, Hirotaka Iwaki, Nicholas Johnson, Sara Bandres-Ciga, Luigi Ferrucci, Faraz Faghri, Andrew B. Singleton, and Mike A. Nalls. "Virus Exposure and Neurodegenerative Disease Risk across National Biobanks." *Neuron*, 111, no. 7 (2023): 1086–93.

Lewis, Talia. "Working Definition of Ableism." *Talila A. Lewis* (blog), January 1, 2022. https://www.talilalewis.com/blog/working-definition-of-ableism-january-2022-update.

Líndal, E., S. Bergmann, S. Thorlacius, and J. G. Stefánsson. "Anxiety Disorders: A Result of Long-Term Chronic Fatigue—The Psychiatric Characteristics of the Sufferers of Iceland Disease." *Acta Neurologica Scandinavia* 96, no. 4 (1997): 158–62.

Liptan, G. L. "Fascia: A Missing Link in Our Understanding of the Pathology of Fibromyalgia." *Journal of Bodywork and Movement Therapies* 14, no. 1 (2010): 3–12.

Lladós, Gemma, Marta Massanella, Roser Coll-Fernández, Raúl Rodríguez, Electra Hernández, Giuseppe Lucente, Cristina López, et al.; Germans Trias Long-COVID Unit Group. "Vagus Nerve Dysfunction in the Post-COVID-19 Condition: A Pilot Cross-Sectional Study." *Clinical Microbiology and Infection* 30, no. 4 (2024): 515–21.

Lock, Margaret. "Comprehending the Body in the Era of the Epigenome." *Current Anthropology* 56, no. 2 (2015): 151–297.

Lock, Margaret, and Vinh-Kim Nguyen. *An Anthropology of Biomedicine*. Wiley-Blackwell, 2010.

Lowe, Abigail E., Kelly K. Dineen, and Seema Mohapatra. "Structural Discrimination in Pandemic Policy: Essential Protections for Essential Workers." *Journal of Law, Medicine, & Ethics* 50, no. 1 (2022): 67–75.

Lowenstein, Fiona. "We Need to Talk about What Coronavirus Recoveries Look Like: They're a Lot More Complicated Than Most People Realize." *New York Times*, April 13, 2020. https://www.nytimes.com/2020/04/13/opinion/coronavirus-recovery.html.

Lunden, Jennifer. *American Breakdown: Our Ailing Nation, My Body's Revolt, and the Nineteenth-Century Woman Who Brought Me Back to Life*. Harper Wave, 2023.

Manderson, L., N. Burke, and A. Wahlberg. *Viral Loads: Anthropologies of Urgency in the Time of COVID-19*. UCL Press, 2022.

Manderson, Lenore, and Ayo Wahlberg. "Chronic Living in a Communicable World." *Medical Anthropology* 39, no. 5 (2020): 428–39.

Manly, Jennifer J., Richard N. Jones, Kenneth M. Langa, Lindsay H. Ryan, Deborah A. Levine, Ryan McCammon, Steven G. Heeringa, and David Weir. "Estimating the Prevalence of Dementia and Mild Cognitive Impairment in the US: The 2016 Health and Retirement Study Harmonized Cognitive Assessment Protocol Project." *JAMA Neurology* 79, no. 12 (2022): 1242–49.

Marcus, Greil. "ONE STEP BACK; Where Are the Elixirs of Yesteryear When We Hurt?" *New York Times*, January 26, 1998. https://www.nytimes.com/1998/01/26/arts/one-step-back-where-are-the-elixirs-of-yesteryear-when-we-hurt.html.

Marinacci, A. A., and K. O. Von Hagen. "The Value of the Electromyogram in the Diagnosis of Iceland Disease." *Electromyography* 5 (1965): 241–51.

Maybin, Jacqueline A., Marianne Watters, Bethan Rowley, Catherine A. Walker, Gemma C. Sharp, and Alexandra Alvergne. "COVID-19 and

Abnormal Uterine Bleeding: Potential Associations and Mechanisms." *Clinical Science* 138, no. 4 (2024): 153–71.

McEvedy, Colin P., and A. W. Beard. "Royal Free Epidemic of 1955: A Reconsideration." *British Medical Journal* 1 (1970): 7–11.

McEwen, Bruce S. "Stress, Adaptation, and Disease: Allostasis and Allostatic Load." *Annals of the New York Academy of Sciences* 840 (1998): 33–44.

Mendenhall, Emily. "Long COVID and the Rise of Digital Patient Activism." *Current History* 124, no. 858 (2025): 9–14.

———. "Long Covid Politics and Activism." *Lancet* 404, no. 10448 (2024): 112–13.

———. *Rethinking Diabetes: Entanglements with Trauma, Poverty, and HIV.* Cornell University Press, 2019.

———. *Syndemic Suffering: Social Distress, Depression, and Diabetes among Mexican Immigrant Women.* Routledge, 2012.

———. *Unmasked: COVID, Community, and the Case of Okoboji.* Vanderbilt University Press, 2022.

Mendenhall, Emily, and Kenton Kaplan. "The 'Brain Fog' of Long COVID Is a Serious Medical Issue That Needs More Attention." *Scientific American*, May 12, 2023. https://www.scientificamerican.com/article/the-brain-fog-of-long-covid-is-a-serious-medical-issue-that-needs-more-attention/.

Merz, Waltraut M., Rebecca Fischer-Betz, Kerstin Hellwig, Georg Lamprecht, and Ulrich Gembruch. "Pregnancy and Autoimmune Disease." *Deutsches Ärzteblatt International* 119, no. 9 (2022): 145–56.

Miller, William R., and Martin E. Seligman. "Depression and Learned Helplessness in Man." *Journal of Abnormal Psychology* 84, no. 3 (1975): 228–38.

Mingus, Mia. "Access Intimacy: The Missing Link." *Leaving Evidence* (blog), May 5, 2011. https://leavingevidence.wordpress.com/2011/05/05/access-intimacy-the-missing-link/.

Miserandino, Christine. "The Spoon Theory." *But You Don't Look Sick*, 2003. https://butyoudontlooksick.com/articles/written-by-christine/the-spoon-theory/.

Mitchell, S. Weir. *Wear and Tear; or Hints for the Overworked.* J. B. Lippincott, 1871.

Mulligan, Jessica, and Heide Castañeda. *Unequal Coverage: The Experience of Health Care Reform in the United States.* NYU Press, 2017.

Murray, Polly. *The Widening Circle: A Lyme Disease Pioneer Tells Her Story.* St. Martin's Press, 1996.

Murray, Stephen O., and Kenneth W. Payne. "The Social Classification of AIDS in American Epidemiology." In *The AIDS Pandemic: A Global Emergency*, edited by Ralph Bolton. Gordon and Breach, 1989.

Musser, John H., and O. A. Kelly. *A Handbook of Practical Treatment*. 1912.

Myers, Neely. *Breaking Points: Youth Mental Health Crises and How We All Can Help*. University of California Press, 2024.

National Institutes of Health. "The Dangers of Polypharmacy and the Case for Deprescribing in Older Adults." National Institute of Aging, August 24, 2021. https://www.nia.nih.gov/news/dangers-polypharmacy-and-case-deprescribing-older-adults.

Navarro, Lygia. "Black and Unbelieved: A Conversation with Filmmaker Chimère Sweeney." *The Sick Times*, June 4, 2024. https://thesicktimes.org/2024/06/04/black-and-unbelieved-a-conversation-with-filmmaker-chimere-sweeney/.

Nezhat, Camran, Farr Nezhat, and Ceana Nezhat. "Endometriosis: Ancient Disease, Ancient Treatments." *Fertility and Sterility* 98, no. 6 Suppl. (2012): S1–62.

Nichter, Mark. "Idioms of Distress Revisited." *Culture, Medicine, and Psychiatry* 34, no. 2 (2010): 401–16.

O'Brien, Kelly K., Ahmed M. Bayoumi, Carol Strike, Nancy L. Young, and Aileen M. Davis. "Exploring Disability from the Perspective of Adults Living with HIV/AIDS: Development of a Conceptual Framework." *Health and Quality of Life Outcomes* 6, no. 76 (2008): 1–11.

O'Rourke, Meghan. *The Invisible Kingdom: Reimagining Chronic Illness*. Riverhead Books, 2022.

———. "A New Name, and Wider Recognition, for Chronic Fatigue Syndrome." *New Yorker*, February 27, 2015. https://www.newyorker.com/tech/annals-of-technology/chronic-fatigue-syndrome-iom-report.

Packard, Randall, Peter J. Brown, Ruth L. Berkelman, and Howard Frumkin. *Emerging Illnesses and Society: Negotiating the Public Health Agenda*. Johns Hopkins University Press, 2004.

———. "Introduction / Emerging Illnesses as Social Process." In *Emerging Illnesses and Society: Negotiating the Public Health Agenda*, edited by Randall Packard, Peter J. Brown, Ruth L. Berkelman, and Howard Frumkin. Johns Hopkins University Press, 2004.

Parish, J. Gordon. "Early Outbreaks of 'Epidemic Neuromyasthenia.'" *Postgraduate Medical Journal* 54 (1978): 711–17.

Parthasarathy, Geetha, Melissa B. Pattison, and Cecily C. Midkiff. "The FGF/ FGFR System in the Microglial Neuroinflammation with *Borrelia burgdorferi*: Likely Intersectionality with Other Neurological Conditions." *Journal of Neuroinflammation* 20, no. 1 (2023): 10.

Patterson, David, and Gerald P. Pyle. "The Diffusion of Influenza in Sub-Saharan Africa during the 1918–1919 Pandemic." *Social Science and Medicine* 17 (1983): 1299–1307.

Pellew, R. A. "A Clinical Description of a Disease Resembling Poliomyelitis, Seen in Adelaide, 1949–1951." *Medical Journal of Australia* 1, no. 26 (1951): 944–46.

Perego, Elisa, Felicity Callard, Laurie Stras, Barbara Melville-Jóhannesson, Rachel Pope, and Nisreen A. Alwan. "Why the Patient-Made Term 'Long Covid' Is Needed." *Wellcome Open Research* 5, no. 224 (2020): 224.

Perlis, Roy H., Mauricio Santillana, Katherine Ognyanova, Alauna Safarpour, Kristin Lunz Trujillo, Matthew D. Simonson, Jon Green, et al. "Prevalence and Correlates of Long COVID Symptoms among US Adults." *JAMA Network Open* 5, no. 10 (2022): e2238804.

Phillips, Howard. *Black October. The Impact of the Spanish Influenza Epidemic of 1918 on South Africa*. Government Printer, 1990.

———. *In a Time of Plague: Memories of the 'Spanish' Flu Epidemic of 1918 in South Africa*. Van Riebeeck Society, 2018.

Phillips, Howard, and David Killingray. *The Spanish Influenza Pandemic of 1918– 1919: New Perspectives*. Routledge, 2003.

Pons-Estel, Guillermo J., Graciela S. Alarcón, Lacie Scofield, Leslie Reinlib, and Glinda S. Cooper. "Understanding the Epidemiology and Progression of Systemic Lupus Erythematosus." *Seminars in Arthritis and Rheumatism* 39, no. 4 (2010): 257–68.

Premraj, Lavienraj, Nivedha V. Kannapadi, Jack Briggs, Stella M. Seal, Denise Battaglini, Jonathon Fanning, Jacky Suen, Chiara Robba, John Fraser, and Sung-Min Cho. "Mid and Long-Term Neurological and Neuropsychiatric Manifestations of Post-COVID-19 Syndrome: A Meta-analysis." *Journal of the Neurological Sciences* 434 (2022): 120162.

Price, Margaret. "The Bodymind Problem and the Possibilities of Pain." *Hypatia* 30, no. 1 (2015): 268–284.

Prior, Ryan. *Forgotten Plague*. Documentary film. Reel Picture, 2015.

———. *The Long Haul: How Long Covid Survivors Are Revolutionizing Healthcare.* MIT Press, 2024.

Proal, Amy, and Michael VanElzakker. "Long COVID or Post-Acute Sequelae of COVID-19 (PASC): An Overview of Biological Factors That May Contribute to Persistent Symptoms." *Frontiers in Microbiology* 12 (2021): 698169.

Pryma, Jane. "'Even My Sister Says I'm Acting Like a Crazy to Get a Check': Race, Gender, and Moral Boundary-Work in Women's Claims of Disabling Chronic Pain." *Social Science and Medicine* 181 (2017): 66–73.

Putnam Jacobi, Mary. *Essays on Hysteria, Brain-Tumor, and Some Other Cases of Nervous Disease,* 1888. [Quoted in Shorter. *From Paralysis to Fatigue: A History of Psychosomatic Illness in the Modern Era.* Free Press, 1992, 223–24.]

———. "Hysterical Fever." *Neurological Section of the Academy of Medicine* April (1890).

———. *The Question of Rest for Women during Menstruation.* G. P. Putnam's Sons, 1877.

Raffety, Erin. *From Inclusion to Justice: Disability, Ministry, and Congregational Leadership.* Baylor University Press, 2022.

Raffety, Erin, and Emma Worrall. "Yo-Yo Hope, 'Symptom Talk,' and the Courage *Not* to Be Well: A Practical Theology of Chronic Illness, Long Covid, and Hope." In *Disability Theology and Eschatology: Hope, Justice, and Flourishing,* edited by Preston McDaniel Hill and Aaron Davis. Bloomsbury, 2025.

Ramanujan, Krishna. "Immune T Cells Become Exhausted in Chronic Fatigue Syndrome Patients." *Cornell Chronicle,* December 3, 2025. https://news .cornell.edu/stories/2024/12/immune-t-cells-become-exhausted-chronic-fatigue-syndrome-patients.

Ramsay, Melvin. "'Epidemic Neuromyasthenia' 1955–1978." *Postgraduate Medical Journal* 54 (1978): 718–21.

———. "Hysteria and 'Royal Free Disease.'" *British Medical Journal* 2, no. 5469 (1965): 1062.

———. *Myalgic Encephalomyelitis and Postviral Fatigue States: The Saga of Royal Free Disease* (originally titled *Postviral Fatigue Syndrome: The Saga of Royal Free Disease*). Gower Medical Publishing, 1986.

Ravenhold, R. T. "Encephalitis Lethargica." In *A World History of Human Disease,* edited by Kenneth Kiple. Cambridge University Press, 1993.

Rawls, William. *Unlocking Lyme: Myths, Truths, and Practical Solutions for Chronic Lyme Disease.* FirstDoNoHarm Publishing, 2017.

Raz, Mical, and Doron Dorfman. "Bans on COVID-19 Mask Requirements vs Disability Accommodations." *JAMA Health Forum* 2, no. 8 (2021): e211912.

Rehmeyer, Julie, and David Tuller. "Getting It Wrong on Chronic Fatigue Syndrome." *New York Times*, March 18, 2017. https://www.nytimes.com/2017/03/18/opinion/sunday/getting-it-wrong-on-chronic-fatigue-syndrome.html.

Reynolds, Matt. "They Never Officially Had COVID-19. Months Later They're Living in Hell." *Wired*, November 9, 2020. https://www.wired.co.uk/article/coronavirus-long-haulers-negative-tests-covid-19.

Rivera-Núñez, Zorimar, Manuel E. Jimenez, Benjamin F. Crabtree, Diane Hill, Maria B. Pellerano, Donita Devance, Myneka Macenat, Daniel Lima, Marsha Gordon, et al. "Experiences of Black and Latinx Health Care Workers in Support Roles during the COVID-19 Pandemic: A Qualitative Study." *PLoS One* 17, no. 1 (2022): e0262606.

Roberts, Melissa H., and Esther Erdei. "Comparative United States Autoimmune Disease Rates for 2010–2016 by Sex, Geographic Region, and Race." *Autoimmunity Reviews* 19, 1 (2020): 102423.

Rogers, Emily Lim. "Illness, Endurance, and Proximities of AIDS Activism." *Feminist Formations* 35, no. 3 (2023): 166.

———. "The Lapsed Ethnographer: Toward Foggy Fieldwork." Edtors' Forum: Theorizing the Contemporary. *Fieldsights*, September 6, 2022. https://culanth.org/fieldsights/the-lapsed-ethnographer-toward-foggy-fieldwork.

———. "Recursive Debility: Symptoms, Patient Activism, and the Incomplete Medicalization of ME/CFS." *Medical Anthropology Quarterly* 36, no. 3 (2022): 412–28.

———. "Staying (at Home) with Brain Fog: 'Un-witting' Patient Activism." *Somatosphere*, October 5, 2020. https://somatosphere.com/2020/staying-home-brain-fog-patient-activism.html/.

Rosenow, E. C., F. R. Heilman, and C. H. Pettet. "Observations on the Epidemic of Polio-Encephalitis in Los Angeles, 1934." *California and Western Medicine* 41, no. 3 (1934): 214–15.

Rosenthal, Thomas C., Barbara A. Majeroni, Richard Pretorious, and Khalid Malik. "Fatigue: An Overview." *American Family Physician* 78, no. 10 (2008): 1173–79.

Sampson, John A. "Peritoneal Endometriosis Due to the Menstrual Dissemination of Endometriosis into the Peritoneal Cavity." *American Journal of Obstetrics and Gynecology* 14, no. 4 (1927): 422–69.

Sapolsky, Robert. *Why Zebras Don't Get Ulcers: The Acclaimed Guide to Stress, Stress-Related Diseases, and Coping.* 3rd ed. Henry Holt, 2004.

Scheper-Hughes, Nancy, and Margaret M. Lock. "The Mindful Body: A Prolegomenon to Future Work in Medical Anthropology." *Medical Anthropology Quarterly* 1, no. 1 (1987): 6–41.

Schuster, David G. *Neurasthenic Nation: America's Search for Health, Happiness, and Comfort, 1869–1920.* Rutgers University Press, 2011.

Seligman, Martin. "Learned Helplessness." *Annual Review of Medicine* 23 (1972): 407–12.

Shackelford, Monica, Thomas Farley, and Cheryl Vines. "A Comparison of Women and Men with Spinal Cord Injury." *Nature* 36 (1998): 337–39.

Sharif, Kassem, Abdulla Watad, Nicola Luigi Bragazzi, Michael Lichtbroun, Mariano Martini, Carlo Perricone, Howard Amital, and Yehuda Shoenfeld. "On Chronic Fatigue Syndrome and Nosological Categories." *Clinical Rheumatology* 37, no. 5 (2018): 1161–70.

Sharma, C., and J. Bayry. "High Risk of Autoimmune Diseases after COVID-19." *Nature Reviews of Rheumatology* 19 (2023): 399–400.

Sharpe, Michael. "Psychiatric Management of PVFS." *British Medical Bulletin* 47, no. 4 (1991): 989–1005.

Sharpe, Michael, and Simon Wessely. "Putting the Rest Cure to Rest—Again." *BMJ* 316 (1998): 796.

Shorter, Edward. "Chronic Fatigue in Historical Perspective." In *Ciba Foundation Symposium 173—Chronic Fatigue Syndrome*, edited by Gregory R. Bock and Julie Whelan (Ciba Foundation 1993.) Novartis Foundation Symposia, 2007.

———. *From Paralysis to Fatigue: A History of Psychosomatic Illness in the Modern Era.* Free Press, 1992.

Showalter, Elaine. *Hystories: Hysterical Epidemics and Modern Culture.* Columbia University Press, 1997.

Sigurdsson, Björn, and Kjartan R. Gudmundsson. "Clinical Findings Six Years after Outbreak of Akureyri Disease." *Lancet* 267, no. 6926 (1956): 766–67.

Singer, Merrill. *Anthropology of Infectious Disease.* Left Coast Press, 2015.

Sins Invalid. *Skin, Tooth, and Bone: The Basis of Movement Is Our People.* 2nd ed. Dancer's Group, 2024. https://www.flipcause.com/secure/reward_step2 /OTMxNQ==/65827.

———. "An Unshamed Claim to Beauty in the Face of Invisibility." *Sins Invalid* (blog), accessed June 10, 2024. https://www.sinsinvalid.org/blog/10-principles-of-disability-justice.

Smith, Chimére L. "Doctors Didn't Believe That I Had COVID-19. I Found a Way to Make Them Listen." CNN, October 17, 2022. https://www.cnn .com/2022/10/17/opinions/long-covid-health-care-smith/index.html.

Snowden, Lonnie R., and Jonathan M. Snowden. "Coronavirus Trauma and African Americans' Mental Health: Seizing Opportunities for Transformational Change." *International Journal of Environmental Research and Public Health* 18, no. 7 (2021): 3568.

Sontag, Susan. *Illness as Metaphor and AIDS and Its Metaphors.* Farrar, Strauss and Giroux, 1978.

Spielman, Andrew, Peter J. Krause, and Sam R. Telford III. "Institutional Responses to the Emergence of Lyme Disease and Its Companion Infections in North America / A Public Health Perspective." In *Emerging Illnesses and Society: Negotiating the Public Health Agenda,* edited by Randall Packard, Peter J. Brown, Ruth L. Berkelman, and Howard Frumkin. Johns Hopkins University Press, 2004.

Spinney, Laura. *Pale Rider: The Spanish Flu of 1918 and How It Changed the World.* Public Affairs, 2017.

Steere, Allen C., Jenifer Coburn, and Lisa Glickstein. "The Emergence of Lyme Disease." *Journal of Clinical Investigation* 113, no. 8 (2004): 1093–101.

Stetson, Charlotte Perkins. "The Yellow Wall-Paper." *New England Magazine,* 1892.

Stricker, Raphael, and Lorraine Johnson. "The Lyme Disease Chronicles, Continued: Chronic Lyme Disease: In Defense of the Patient Enterprise." *Federation of American Societies for Experimental Biology* 24 (2010): 4632–33.

Tampa, Mircea, Ioan Sarbu, C. Matei, V. Benea, and S. R. Georgescu. "Brief History of Syphilis." *Journal of Medicine and Life* 7 (2014): 4–10.

Tasca, Cecilia, Mariangela Rapetti, Mauro Giovanni Carta, and Bianca Fadda. "Women and Hysteria in the History of Mental Health." *Clinical Practice & Epidemiology in Mental Health* 8 (2012): 110–19.

Taylor, Ruth. "A Study of Neurasthenia at the National Hospital for the Relief and Cure of the Paralysed and Epileptic, Queen Square, London, 1870–1932." *British Journal of Psychiatry* 179, no. 6 (2001): 550–57.

Taylor, Sunaura. *Disabled Ecologies: Lessons from a Wounded Desert.* University of California Press, 2024.

Tilt, Edward John. *On Diseases of Menstruation and Ovarian Inflammation.* Samuel S. and William Wood, 1851.

Timmermans, Stefan, and Marc Berg. *The Gold Standard: The Challenge of Evidence-Based Medicine and Standardization in Health Care.* Temple University Press, 2003.

Tonks, Alison. "Lyme Wars." *Infectious Diseases* 335, no. 7626 (2007): 910–12.

Tuller, David. "An Open Letter to The Lancet, Again." *Virology Blog*, February 10, 2016. https://virology.ws/2016/02/10/open-letter-lancet-again/.

———. "Reexamining Chronic Fatigue Syndrome Research and Treatment Policy." *Health Affairs Blog*, February 4, 2016. https://www.healthaffairs.org/content/forefront/reexamining-chronic-fatigue-syndrome-research-and-treatment-policy.

———. "Trial by Error: Open Letter to The Lancet, Version 3.0." *Virology Blog*, August 13, 2018. https://virology.ws/2018/08/13/trial-by-error-open-letter-to-the-lancet-version-3-0/.

———. "Trial by Error: The Troubling Case of the PACE Chronic Fatigue Syndrome Study." *Virology Blog*, October 21, 2015. https://virology.ws/2015/10/21/trial-by-error-i/.

———. "Worse Than Disease: Curing Chronic Fatigue." *UnDark*, October 27, 2016. https://undark.org/2016/10/27/chronic-fatigue-graded-exercise-pace/.

Underhill, Rosemary, and Rosemarie Baillod. "Myalgic Encephalomyelitis/Chronic Fatigue Syndrome: Organic Disease or Psychosomatic Illness? A Re-Examination of the Royal Free Epidemic of 1955." *Medicina* 57, no. 1 (2021): 12.

van der Feltz-Cornelis, Christina Maria, Fidan Turk, Jennifer Sweetman, Kamlesh Khunti, Mark Gabbay, Jessie Shepherd, Hugh Montgomery, et al. "Prevalence of Mental Health Conditions and Brain Fog in People with Long COVID: A Systematic Review and Meta-analysis." *General Hospital Psychiatry* 88 (2024): 10–22.

Van der Kolk, Bessel. *The Body Keeps the Score: Brain, Mind, and Body in the Healing of Trauma.* Penguin Books, 2015.

Van Deusen, E. H. "Observations on a Form of Nervous Prostration, (Neurasthenia) Culminating in Insanity." *American Journal of Insanity* 25, no. 4 (1869): 445–61.

VanElzakker, Michael B. "Chronic Fatigue Syndrome from Vagus Nerve Infection: A Psychoneuroimmunological Hypothesis." *Medical Hypotheses* 81, no. 3 (2013): 414–23.

Veyrié, Axel, Antoine Netter, Xavier Carcopino, Laura Miquel, Aubert Agostini, and Blandine Courbiere. "Endometriosis and Pregnancy: The Illusion of Recovery." *PLoS One* 17, no. 11 (2022): e0272828.

Vojdani, Aristo, Elroy Vojdani, Evan Saidara, and Michael Maes. "Persistent SARS-CoV-2 Infection, EBV, HHV-6 and Other Factors May Contribute to Inflammation and Autoimmunity in Long COVID." *Viruses* 15, no. 2 (2023): 400.

Wahlberg, Ayo. "Serious Disease as Kinds of Living." In *Contested Categories: Life Sciences in Society*, edited by S. Bauer and A. Wahlberg. Ashgate, 2009.

Wang, Siwen, Luwei Quan, Jorge E. Chavarro, Natalie Slopen, Laura D. Kubzansky, Karestan C. Koenen, Jae Hee Kang, et al. "Associations of Depression, Anxiety, Worry, Perceived Stress, and Loneliness Prior to Infection with Risk of Post–COVID-19 Conditions." *JAMA Psychiatry* 79, no. 11 (2022): 1081–91.

Ware, Norma. "Society, Mind and Body in Chronic Fatigue Syndrome: An Anthropological View." In *Ciba Foundation Symposium 173—Chronic Fatigue Syndrome*, edited by Gary R. Bock and Julie Whelan. (Ciba Foundation 1993.) Novartis Foundation Symposia, 2007.

———. "Suffering and the Social Construction of Illness: The Delegitimation of Illness Experience in Chronic Fatigue Syndrome." *Medical Anthropology Quarterly* 6 (1992): 347–61.

———. "Toward a Model of Social Course in Chronic Illness: The Example of Chronic Fatigue Syndrome." *Culture, Medicine and Psychiatry* 23 (1999): 303–31.

Ware, Norma, and Arthur Kleinman. "Culture and Somatic Experience: The Social Course of Illness in Neurasthenia and Chronic Fatigue Syndrome." *Psychosomatic Medicine* 54, no. 5 (1992): 546–60.

Webster, Richard. *Freud, Charcot and Hysteria: Lost in the Labyrinth.* Self-published, 2004.

Weintraub, Pamela. *Cure Unknown: Inside the Lyme Epidemic.* St. Martin's Griffin, 2008.

Wendell, Susan. *The Rejected Body: Feminist Philosophical Reflections on Disability.* Routledge, 1996.

———. "Unhealthy Disabled: Treating Chronic Illnesses as Disabilities." *Hypatia* 16, no. 4 (2001): 17–33.

Wessely, Simon. "The Neuropsychiatry of Chronic Fatigue Syndrome," *Ciba Foundation Symposium 173—Chronic Fatigue Syndrome,* edited by Gregory R. Bock & Julie Whelan. (Ciba Foundation 1993.) Novartis Foundation Symposia, 2007.

———. "Old Wine in New Bottles: Neurasthenia and 'ME.'" *Psychological Medicine* 20 (1990): 35–53.

Wessely, Simon, and Anthony J. Cleare. "Chronic Fatigue Syndrome." In *Encyclopedia of Stress,* edited by George Fink. Academic Press, 2000.

Wessely, S., and R. Powell. "Fatigue Syndromes: A Comparison of Chronic 'Postviral' Fatigue with Neuromuscular and Affective Disorders." *Journal of Neurology, Neurosurgery, and Psychiatry* 52, no. 8 (1989): 940–48.

Whitaker, Robert C., Tracy Dearth-Wesley, Allison N. Herman, Amy E. Block, Mary Howard Holderness, Nicholas A. Waring, and J. Michael Oakes. "The Interaction of Adverse Childhood Experiences and Gender as Risk Factors for Depression and Anxiety Disorders in US Adults: A Cross-sectional Study." *BMC Public Health* 21, no. 2078 (2021).

White, P. D., Kim Goldsmith, A. L. Johnson, Trudie Chalder, Michael Sharpe, and PACE Trial Management Group. "Recovery from Chronic Fatigue Syndrome after Treatments Given in the PACE Trial." *Psychological Medicine* 43, no. 10 (2013): 2227–35.

White, P. D., Kim A. Goldsmith, A. L. Johnson, L. Potts, R. Walwyn, J. C. DeCesare, H. L. Baber, et al.; PACE Trial Management Group. "Comparison of Adaptive Pacing Therapy, Cognitive Behaviour Therapy, Graded Exercise Therapy, and Specialist Medical Care for Chronic Fatigue Syndrome (PACE): A Randomised Trial." *Lancet* 377, no. 9768 (2011): 823–36.

Wilson, Elizabeth. *Gut Feminism.* Duke University Press, 2015.

———. *Psychosomatic: Feminism and the Neurological Body.* Duke University Press, 2004.

Yoon, Ji-Hai, Na-Huyn Park, Ye-Eun Kang, Yo-Chan Ahn, Eun-Jung lee, and Ghang-Gue Son. "The Demographic Features of Fatigue in the General

Population Worldwide: A Systematic Review and Meta-analysis." *Frontiers in Public Health* 11 (2023).

Yong, Ed. *I Contain Multitudes: The Microbes within Us and a Grander View of Life.* Ecco, 2016.

———. "Reporting on Long Covid Taught Me to Be a Better Journalist." *New York Times*, December 11, 2023. https://www.nytimes.com/2023/12/11/opinion/long-covid-reporting-lessons.html.

Young, Allan. *The Harmony of Illusions: Inventing Post-Traumatic Stress Disorder.* Princeton University Press, 1995.

Zabiliūtė, Emilija, and Hannah McNeilly. "Relational Chronicities: Kinship, Care, and Ethics of Responsibility." *Anthropology & Medicine* 30, no. 3 (2023): 171–83.

Zanza, Christian, Tatsiana Romenskaya, Alice Chiara Manetti, Francesco Franceschi, Raffaele La Russa, Giuseppe Bertozzi, Aniello Maiese, et al. "Cytokine Storm in COVID-19: Immunopathogenesis and Therapy." *Medicina* (Kaunas) 58, no. 2 (2022): 144.

Zhang, Li. *Anxious China: Inner Revolution and Politics of Psychotherapy.* University of California Press, 2020.

Zheng, Y. P., K. M. Lin, J. Yamamoto, D. C. Zhang, G. Nakasaki, and H. K. Feng. "Neurasthenia in Chinese Students and Visiting Scholars in the United States." *Psychiatric Annals* 22 (1992): 173–87.

Index

173–76; structural silencing and, 13–17. *See also* memory

chronic stress, 102–3

Ciba Foundation, 59–63, 65

Clearing the Fog (Jackson), 174–75

Cleghorn, Elinor, 38

COBRA, 148

cognitive behavioral therapy (CBT), 64–65. *See also* PACE Trial

complex chronic health conditions: clinicians and treatment approaches to, 7–8; disability consciousness and, 125–27; glossary for, xi–xvi (*see also specific conditions*); as "illnesses you have to fight to get," 76–77; impact of long COVID on, 9–12, 179; misogynies and, 10–11, 113; post-viral conditions and, 42–47; reimagining care for, 166–67, 180–84; research methods and, ix–x, 18–22; trauma and, 17–18. *See also* chronic living

complex regional pain syndrome (CRPS), xiii

conversion hysteria, 30. *See also* functional neurological disorder (FND)

Coombs, Krista, 127

cough of Perinthus, 42

COVID-19 Longhauler Advocacy Project, 143

COVID-19 pandemic: anti-Asian violence and, 120; "China virus" and, 43; cytokine storms and, 99, 103; Lyme disease and, 85. *See also* long COVID

credibility economy, 155–57

Crenshaw, Kimberleé, 20–21

crip, use of term, xi

crip time, 121

Crowded Out (Kenworthy), 150

crowdfunding, 150

Cultural Revolution. *See shenjing shuairuo* (neurasthenia)

cytokines, 99, 103

Davids, JD, 137–39, 140, 176

Davis, Hanna, 142

deep memory, 57

dementia, 51, 74, 115, 119

dengue, 115

depression: chronic fatigue syndrome (CFS) and, 64–66; COVID-19 and, 110; endometriosis and, 91; learned helplessness and, 64–65; Lyme disease and, 76–77, 79; ME/CFS and, 119; neurasthenia and, 36, 53–62; trauma and, 96

Diagnostic and Statistical Manual (DSM-III), 27, 57–58

Diagnostic and Statistical Manual (DSM-IV), 196n29

Diagnostic and Statistical Manual (DSM-V), 27

Diedrich, Lisa, 136–37

disability, construct of, 125–27

disability justice movement, xi, 11, 128, 139–42. *See also* AIDS activism; embodied health movements

disability rights movements, 127–28

Disabled Ecologies (Taylor), 100–101

Divided Bodies (Dumes), 14, 77, 83, 93

Dorfman, Doron, 127, 140

Dumes, Abigail A., 14, 77, 81, 83, 93

Dumit, Joe, 76–77

dysautonomia, xiii, 15–16, 76–77, 78, 104

dystonia, xiii

myalgic encephalomyelitis (ME): definition and classification of, xv, 50–51; Incline Village outbreak (1984) and, 48–52; poliomyelitis and, 45–46; Royal Free Hospital outbreak (London, 1955) and, xv, 46–47, 50

myalgic encephalomyelitis/chronic fatigue syndrome (ME/CFS): antecedents of, 48–52; definition and classification of, xv, 63–64; embodied health movements and, 132–33, 134–40; Jo's story and, 116–21, 176; manifestation of fatigue in, 121–24; vagus nerve and, 103–4

#MyDisabledLifeIsWorthy, 145

Myers, Neely, 112–13

National Breast Cancer Coalition, 134

National Center for Complementary and Alternative Medicine, 63

National Health Service (NHS), 71

National Institute of Allergy and Infectious Disease (NIAID), 63

National Institute of Mental Health (NIMH), 63

National Institutes of Health (NIH), xii, 60–63, 69

Nell (research participant), 175–76

neurasthenia: anthropological perspective on, 53–62; definition of, xv; history of, 36–39, 40–41; men and, 37, 38, 40–41; productivity and, 113; in "The Yellow Wall-Paper" (Stetson), 178

Neurasthenic Nation (Schuster), 37

neuroracism, 157–59

The New England Magazine (literary magazine), 178

The New Yorker (magazine), 69

The New York Times (newspaper), 69, 113, 141

The New York Times Sunday Magazine, 134

O'Rourke, Megan, 76

Osler's Web (Johnson), 49, 51

PACE Trial, 66–72, 136

patient activism: disability justice movement and, xi, 11, 128, 139–42; disability rights movements and, 127–28. See also AIDS activism; embodied health movements

Patient-Generated Hypotheses (journal), 142

Patient-Led Research Collaboration (PLRC), 142

people of color: COVID-19 pandemic and, 170–73; dismissal of physical pain and psychological distress of, 34; structural silencing and, 152–54, 156–61. See also Black women

Perego, Elisa, 141, 143

Peter. See Brown, Peter

Peterson, Daniel, 48–50

pharmaceutical industry, 37

Phillips, Howard, 44

pneumonia, 115

poliomyelitis, 45–46

PolyBio Research Foundation, 143–44

post-exertional malaise exacerbation (PEME), 63–65, 66–72, 120–21, 122, 123, 127, 153

postural orthostatic tachycardia syndrome (POTS), xv, 5, 152–53

post-viral conditions, 42–47. See also influenza; long COVID

Sweeney, Chimére L., 145, 160–61, 176
syphilis, 115
systemic exertion intolerance disease
  (SEIM), 69
systemic lupus erythematosus (SLE), xiv,
  97–98, 122, 158–60

Tam. *See* Brand, Tamara (Tam)
Taylor, Sunaura, 100–101
T cells, 104
testimonial injustice, 155–57
Theresa (research participant), 148–50
thresholds metaphor: concept of, 6,
  89–90, 104–5; long COVID and, 6–7;
  Lyme disease and, 84–85; microbiomes and, 101–3; Tam's story and,
  90–92; verifiability and, 88–90, 96
Tilt, Edward, 31
tilt table test, 153
TIME (magazine), 136
Timmermans, Stefan, 82–83
trauma: chronic living and, 168; complex
  chronic health conditions and, 17–18;
  COVID-19 pandemic and, 171–73;
  eating disorders and, 95; hysteria and,
  32–33; long COVID and, 10; neurasthenia and, 56–57; pain without verifiability and, 95–97
traumatic brain injury, 115
Tuller, David, 69–71, 132–33, 136
Ty. *See* Godwin, Ty
type 2 diabetes, 17–18

ulcerative colitis, 98–99
Unrest (documentary film), 118, 121–22

vagus nerve, 103–4
Van Deusen, E. H., 38
VanElzakker, Michael, 143–44
VanElzakker, Mike, 103–4
Verduzco-Gutierrez, Monica, 6–7
verifiability: legitimacy and, 13–14; Tam's
  story and, 90–92, 95–100, 176;
  thresholds metaphor and, 88–90, 96
Virology Blog (website), 69–71
vital essentialism, 56, 58
Voice of the Patient (FDA), 69

Wahlberg, Ayo, 12
Ware, Norma, 52, 53, 62
Watson, Amy, 190n17
weathering, 6, 89, 158
Wei, Hannah, 142
Wendell, Susan, 125
Wessely, Simon, 64–68
West Nile, 115
White, Peter D., 198n78
Why Zebras Don't Get Ulcers (Sapolsky),
  89–90
Willis, Thomas, 29
Wilson, Elizabeth, 27, 41, 95, 101, 104
women of color, 34. *See also* Black women
women's suffrage movements, 41
Woolf, Virginia, 38
Writing at the Margin (Kleinman), 56

"The Yellow Wall-Paper" (Stetson), 178
Yong, Ed, 113
Young, Allan, 57

Zika, 115

Founded in 1893,
UNIVERSITY OF CALIFORNIA PRESS
publishes bold, progressive books and journals
on topics in the arts, humanities, social sciences,
and natural sciences—with a focus on social
justice issues—that inspire thought and action
among readers worldwide.

The UC PRESS FOUNDATION
raises funds to uphold the press's vital role
as an independent, nonprofit publisher, and
receives philanthropic support from a wide
range of individuals and institutions—and from
committed readers like you. To learn more, visit
ucpress.edu/supportus.